We gratefully acknowledge
Dr. Felicien M. Steichen's untiring help
in the editing of this Atlas.
We further thank Dr. Felicien M. Steichen,
Dr. Mark M. Ravitch and the many surgeons
worldwide who have contributed to the
art of stapling in surgery.

We gratefully acknowledge
Dr. Felicien M. Steichen's untiring help
in the editing of this Atlas.
We further thank Dr. Felicien M. Steichen,
Dr. Mark M. Ravitch and the many surgeons
worldwide who have contributed to the
art of stapling in surgery.

Many textbooks and medical papers have been published addressing the use of stapling in surgery; some of these books are listed at the end of this Atlas.

STAPLING TECHNIQUES
GENERAL SURGERY

with Auto Suture® instruments

THIRD EDITION

For further information
please contact:

United States Surgical Corporation
Education Department
150 Glover Ave., Norwalk, CT 06856
1-800-722-USSC

CONTENTS

This publication illustrates some surgical stapling techniques in general surgery. Before using any Auto Suture® surgical stapling instrument, read carefully the current information booklet for that device.

The use of Auto Suture® staplers in
GENERAL SURGERY

The use of Auto Suture® surgical staplers provides significant benefits to the surgeon and his patient.

The instruments have wide application in general surgery facilitating ligation and division, resection, anastomosis, and skin and fascia closure. Flexibility in technique is broad with minimal change required in the surgical approach to most procedures.

The use of the Auto Suture® surgical staplers can significantly reduce operating time, time under anesthesia, blood loss, tissue manipulation and trauma, thereby facilitating postoperative healing. The staplers provide an excellent means of tissue closure prior to resection, reducing tissue handling and intraperitoneal soilage.

The non-crushing "B" shape of the stainless steel staples provides hemostasis, yet permits nutrition to pass through the staple line to the cut edge of the tissue, promoting healing and reducing the possibility of necrosis. The staples are essentially non-reactive to the tissue.

Flexibility in technique is broad. The operator can perform anastomoses end-to-end, end-to-side, side-to-side or with one of the widely used "functional" end-to-end methods.

Edema and inflammation usually associated with manual suturing is significantly reduced as a result of minimal tissue manipulation during the application of the staplers. Anastomoses appear to function sooner than with manual suturing techniques.

The use of Auto Suture® surgical staplers enhances surgery and provides improved patient care.

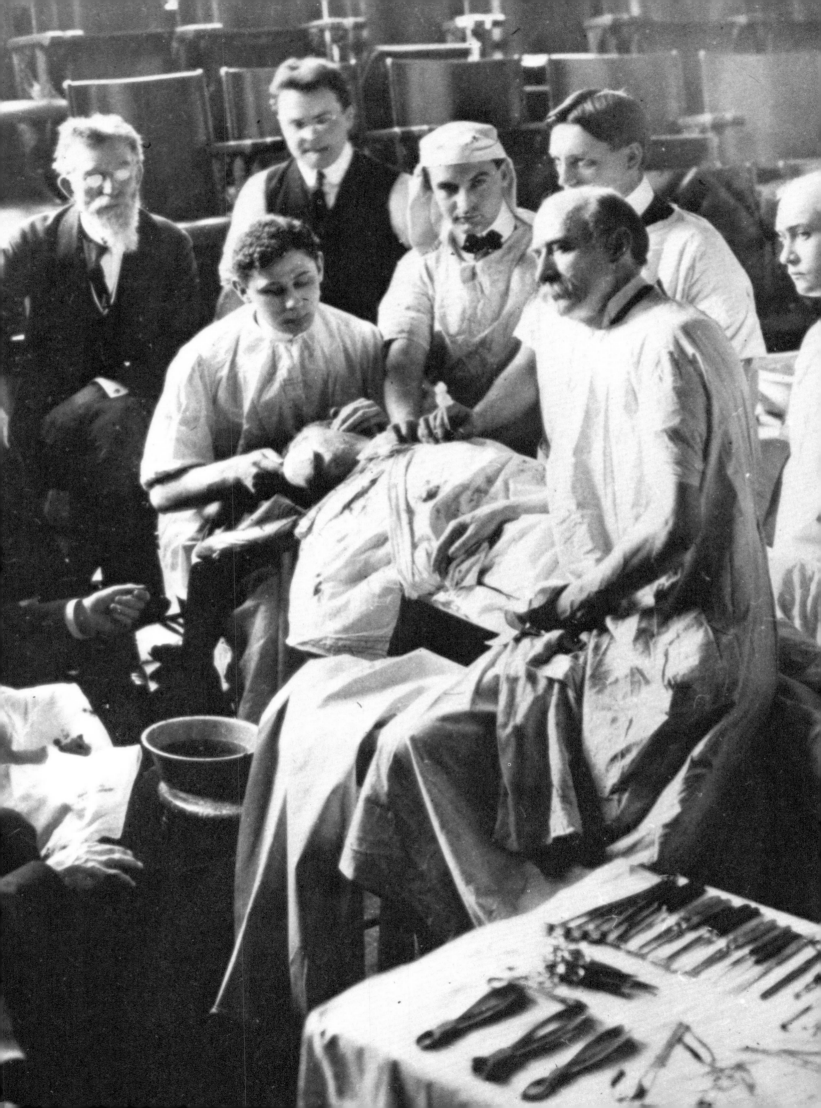

ESOPHAGEAL SURGERY

Esophagogastrectomy

Auto Suture® Instruments Used in an Esophagogastrectomy and Esophagogastrostomy

See Cautions and Contraindications on page 236

INSTRUMENT	CLINICAL APPLICATION
LDS™ Instrument	Ligation and division of the omental vessels and vagus nerves.
TA® 90 Instrument	Closure of the gastric fundus.
GIA™ Instrument	Creation of the gastrotomy. Alternate technique: Anastomosis of the esophagus to the stomach.
EEA™ Instrument or PREMIUM CEEA™ Instrument	Anastomosis of the esophagus to the stomach.
TA® 55 Instrument	Closure of the gastrotomy. Closure of the pyloroplasty incision.
TA® 30 Instrument	Alternate technique: Closure of the esophagus and the gastric stab wound.
DFS™ Instrument and PREMIUM® Skin Stapler	Closure of fascia and skin.

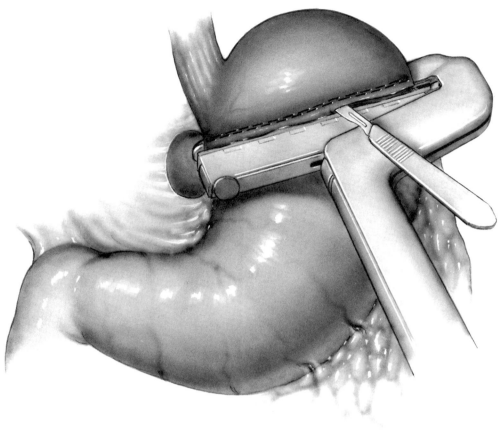

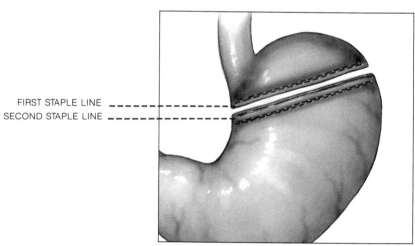

FIRST STAPLE LINE - - - - - - - - - - -
SECOND STAPLE LINE - - - - - - - - - -

The distal esophagus and proximal stomach are mobilized using the LDS™ instrument to ligate and divide the omental vessels, including the left gastric artery, and the vagus nerves.

The gastric fundus is stapled with two applications of the TA® 90 instrument. Following the first application, the TA® 90 instrument is reapplied parallel and distal to the previous staple line. After the second application of the TA® 90 instrument, the stomach is transected between the two double staple lines using the superior edge of the instrument as a cutting guide.

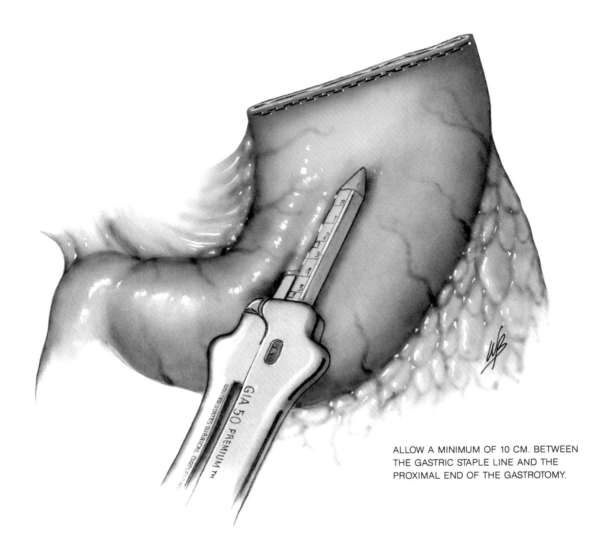

ALLOW A MINIMUM OF 10 CM. BETWEEN
THE GASTRIC STAPLE LINE AND THE
PROXIMAL END OF THE GASTROTOMY.

The GIA™ instrument is used to incise the stomach and secure hemostasis of the cut edges. A 1 cm. stab wound is made into the anterior gastric wall at the level for the gastrotomy. Insert the anvil fork of the GIA™ instrument into the lumen of the stomach and place the cartridge fork on the serosal surface. Close the instrument and fire the staples. Two double staggered staple lines are placed in the gastric wall and the knife blade in the instrument incises the gastric wall between them.

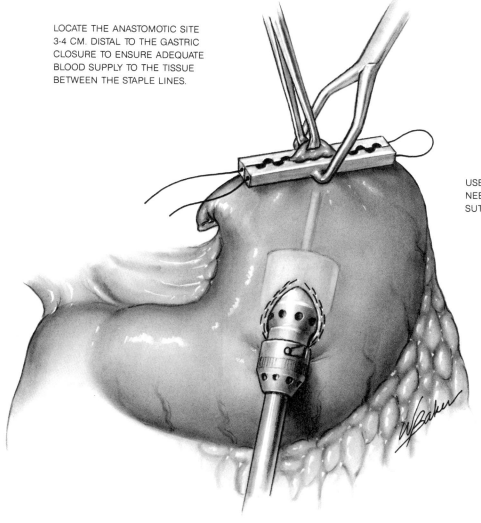

LOCATE THE ANASTOMOTIC SITE 3-4 CM. DISTAL TO THE GASTRIC CLOSURE TO ENSURE ADEQUATE BLOOD SUPPLY TO THE TISSUE BETWEEN THE STAPLE LINES.

USE A SWAGED ON 3″ STRAIGHT NEEDLE WITH A 00 MONOFILAMENT SUTURE FOR THE PURSE STRING.

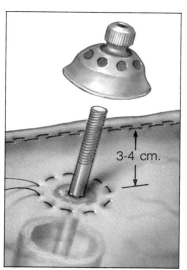

3-4 cm.

Identify the location of the anastomosis 3-4 cm. distal to the stapled gastric closure. With an Allis clamp, grasp all tissue layers of the gastric wall. Apply the purse string instrument around the gastric tissue just beneath the Allis clamp and place a purse string suture. Excise the redundant tissue using the purse string instrument as a cutting guide.

The EEA™ instrument is used to create the anastomosis. Introduce the instrument, without anvil, into the gastric incision. Remove the purse string instrument and pass the center rod through the gastric wall. Open the instrument, tie the purse string suture and place the anvil on the center rod.

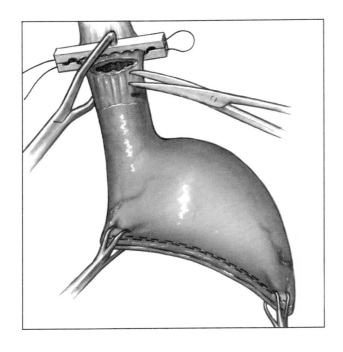

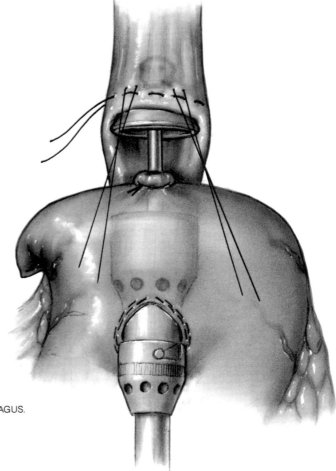

TRACTION ON THE SPECIMEN FACILITATES
INTRODUCTION OF THE ANVIL INTO THE ESOPHAGUS.

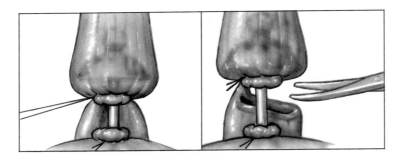

The purse string instrument is placed around the esophagus just proximal to the point of transection. Place a purse string suture and incise the anterior wall of the esophagus on the specimen side using the purse string instrument as a cutting guide. Remove the purse string instrument and place two traction sutures or two Allis clamps on the anterior wall of the proximal esophagus. Introduce the anvil into the esophagus, using traction on the sutures and the specimen to facilitate placement. Tie the purse string suture and transect the posterior wall of the distal esophagus resecting the specimen.

Alternate Technique

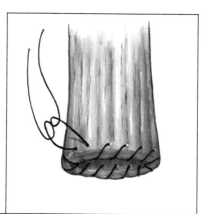

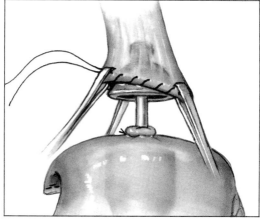

TO FACILITATE INSERTION, PLACE THE POSTERIOR
WALL OF THE ESOPHAGUS OVER THE EDGE OF
THE ANVIL FIRST.

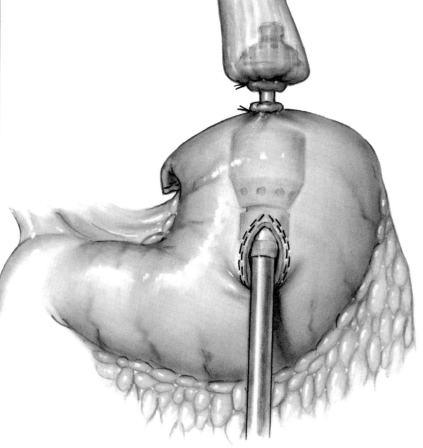

The purse string suture on the esophagus may be
placed manually following complete transection of the
esophagus. Grasp the esophageal edges with three
Allis clamps placed equidistantly. Introduce the anvil
into the esophagus and tie the purse string suture.

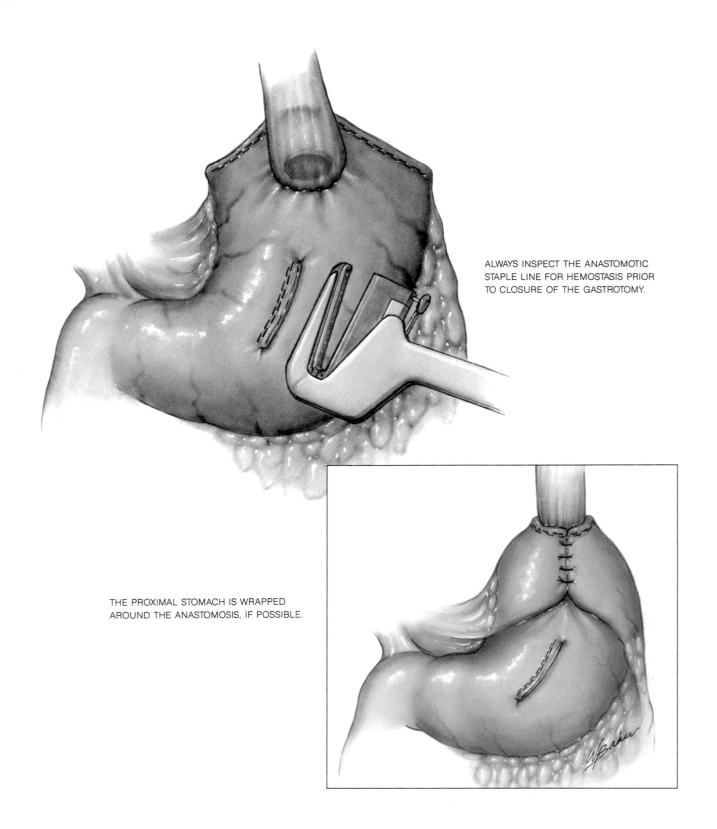

ALWAYS INSPECT THE ANASTOMOTIC
STAPLE LINE FOR HEMOSTASIS PRIOR
TO CLOSURE OF THE GASTROTOMY.

THE PROXIMAL STOMACH IS WRAPPED
AROUND THE ANASTOMOSIS, IF POSSIBLE.

Close the EEA™ instrument and fire the staples.
A circular double staggered row of staples join the
organs and the circular blade in the instrument cuts
a stoma. Open the instrument slightly, place a traction
or figure-of-eight suture around the staple line, lift the
edge of the staple line over the anvil; simultaneously,
gently rotate and remove the instrument.

Check the tissue within the cartridge of the EEA™
instrument for continuity of the purse string sutures
and presence of all tissue layers. Inspect the
anastomotic staple line for hemostasis prior to closing
the gastrotomy with the TA® 55 instrument.

Esophagogastrostomy with Pyloroplasty

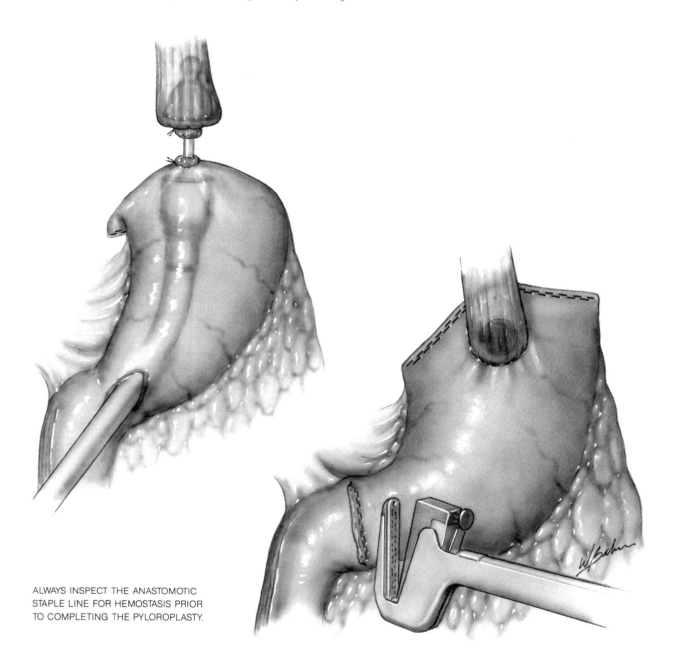

ALWAYS INSPECT THE ANASTOMOTIC
STAPLE LINE FOR HEMOSTASIS PRIOR
TO COMPLETING THE PYLOROPLASTY.

The esophagogastrectomy is performed as previously described.

A Heineke-Mikulicz pyloroplasty incision is made across the pylorus. The incision is initially used as the introduction site for the EEA™ instrument used to perform the esophagogastrostomy. Following completion of the anastomosis and inspection of the staple line for hemostasis, the longitudinal incision is closed transversely with the TA® 55 instrument, completing the pyloroplasty. This procedure may be used for anastomosis just above or at the level of the diaphragm.

End-to-End Anastomosis

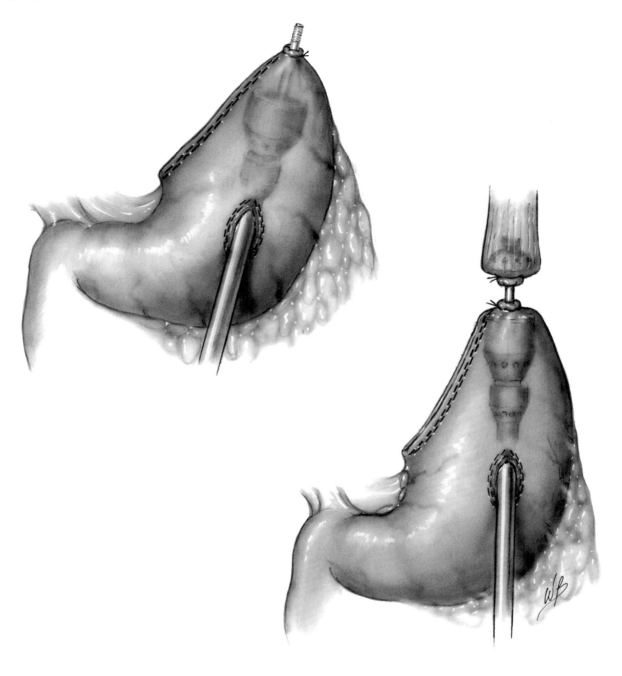

An end-to-end esophagogastrostomy may be performed utilizing the greater curvature corner of the gastric closure. Introduce the EEA™ instrument, without anvil, through the gastrotomy. Excise the corner of the gastric staple line and place a manual purse string suture. Open the EEA™ instrument, advancing the center rod through the opening. Tie the purse string suture and place the anvil on the center rod. Introduce the anvil into the esophagus and tie the purse string suture. Complete the anastomosis as previously described.

Alternate Technique

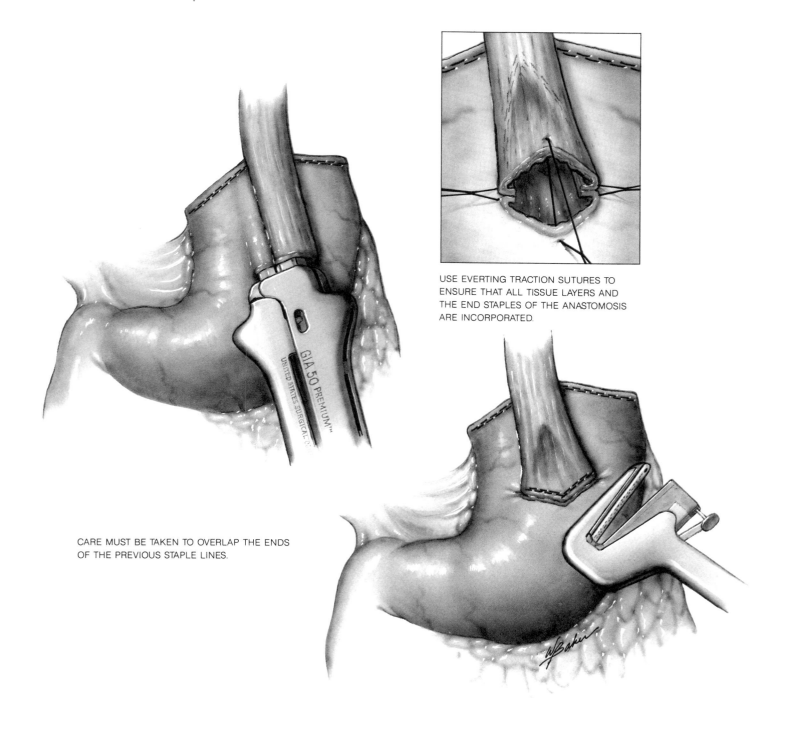

USE EVERTING TRACTION SUTURES TO
ENSURE THAT ALL TISSUE LAYERS AND
THE END STAPLES OF THE ANASTOMOSIS
ARE INCORPORATED.

CARE MUST BE TAKEN TO OVERLAP THE ENDS
OF THE PREVIOUS STAPLE LINES.

The esophagogastrostomy may be performed using
the GIA™ instrument. Make a 1 cm. stab wound into
the anterior gastric wall approximately 8 cm. from the
gastric staple line closure. Insert the anvil fork of the
GIA™ instrument into the lumen of the stomach and
the cartridge fork into the lumen of the esophagus.
Close the instrument †end fire the staples.

Inspect the anastomotic staple lines for hemostasis
prior to closure of the common opening with two
applications of the TA® 30 instrument.

The fascia and skin are closed in the usual manner
with the DFS™ instrument and the PREMIUM® skin
stapler.

Esophagectomy and Reverse Gastric Tube

Auto Suture® Instruments Used in an Esophagectomy and Reverse Gastric Tube with Splenectomy

See Cautions and Contraindications on page 236

INSTRUMENT	CLINICAL APPLICATION
LDS™ Instrument	Ligation and division of the omental and splenic vessels.
GIA™ Instrument	Creation of the reverse gastric tube. Temporary closure and transection of the duodenum for the extended tube.
TA® 55 Instrument	Closure of the esophagus. Alternate technique: Closure of the gastrotomy.
EEA™ Instrument or PREMIUM CEEA™ Instrument	Anastomosis of the esophagus to the gastric tube. Alternate technique: Anastomosis of the stomach to the duodenum.
DFS™ Instrument and PREMIUM® Skin Stapler	Closure of fascia and skin.

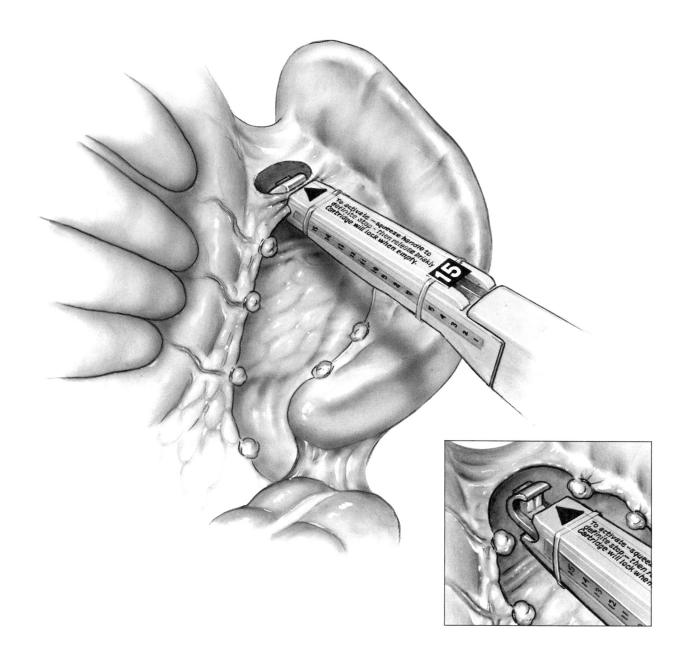

To achieve mobility of the left gastroepiploic vessels, a splenectomy is performed using the LDS™ instrument to ligate and divide the gastrosplenic ligament directly on the splenic capsule. Slip the vessel(s) to be ligated into the jaw of the LDS™ instrument and fire the staples. Simultaneously, two staples ligate the vessel and a knife blade divides the vessel between the staples.

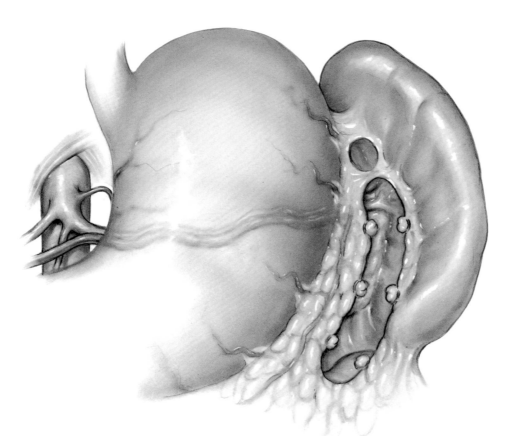

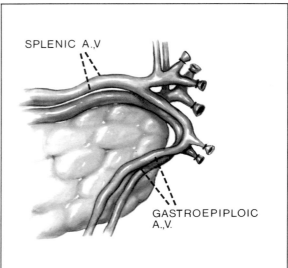

SPLENIC A.,V

GASTROEPIPLOIC A.,V.

The LDS™ instrument is helpful if the splenophrenic, splenorenal and splenocolic ligaments are vascular.

The spleen is elevated and the LDS™ instrument is used to separately ligate and divide the splenic artery and vein.

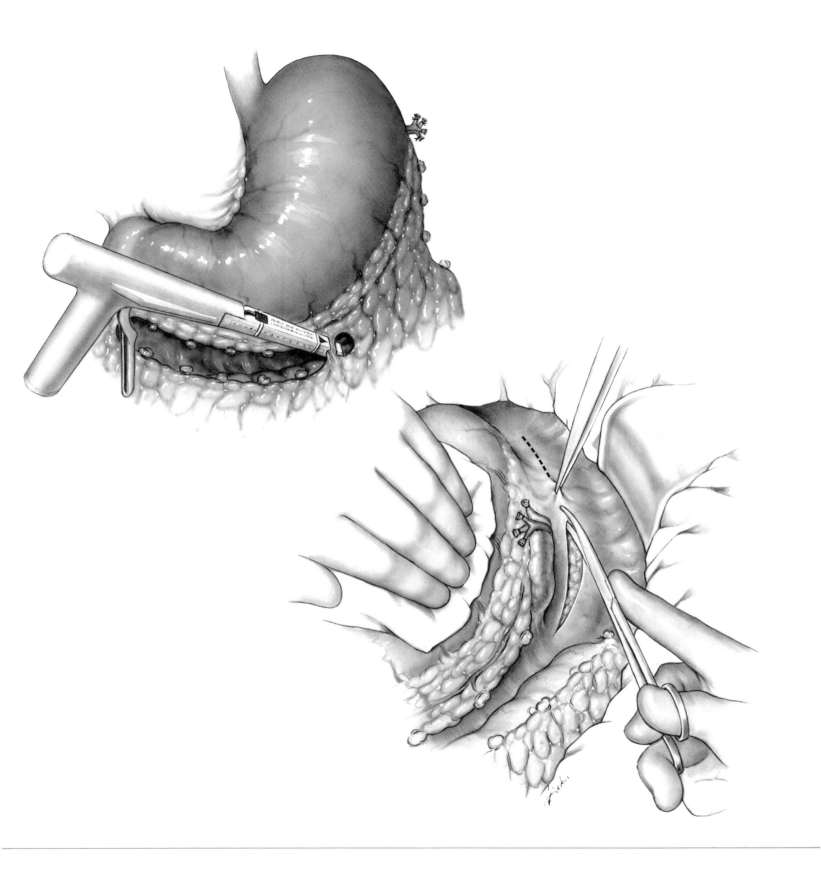

The LDS™ instrument is used to ligate and divide the gastrocolic omentum peripheral to the gastroepiploic vessels.

Prior to creating the gastric tube, the posterior peritoneum is incised and the pancreas is elevated in a medial direction to increase upward mobility.

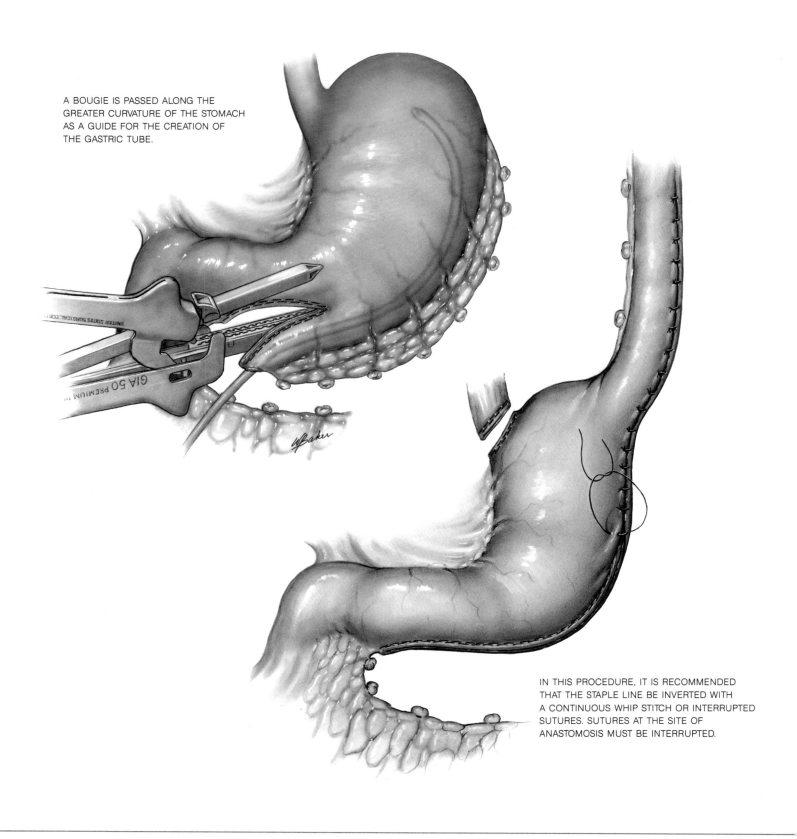

A BOUGIE IS PASSED ALONG THE
GREATER CURVATURE OF THE STOMACH
AS A GUIDE FOR THE CREATION OF
THE GASTRIC TUBE.

IN THIS PROCEDURE, IT IS RECOMMENDED
THAT THE STAPLE LINE BE INVERTED WITH
A CONTINUOUS WHIP STITCH OR INTERRUPTED
SUTURES. SUTURES AT THE SITE OF
ANASTOMOSIS MUST BE INTERRUPTED.

A reverse gastric tube is created using serial applications of the GIA™ instrument. Apply the instrument along the greater curvature of the stomach beginning approximately 2-3 cm. proximal to the pylorus. Reapply the GIA™ instrument until the tube is completed.

The distal esophagus is transected between two applications of the TA® 55 instrument. The second application of the instrument is placed parallel and distal to the first staple line and the superior edge of the instrument is used as a cutting guide.

The anastomosis of the reverse gastric tube to the esophagus is performed manually.

Extended Reverse Gastric Tube – Gavriliu II

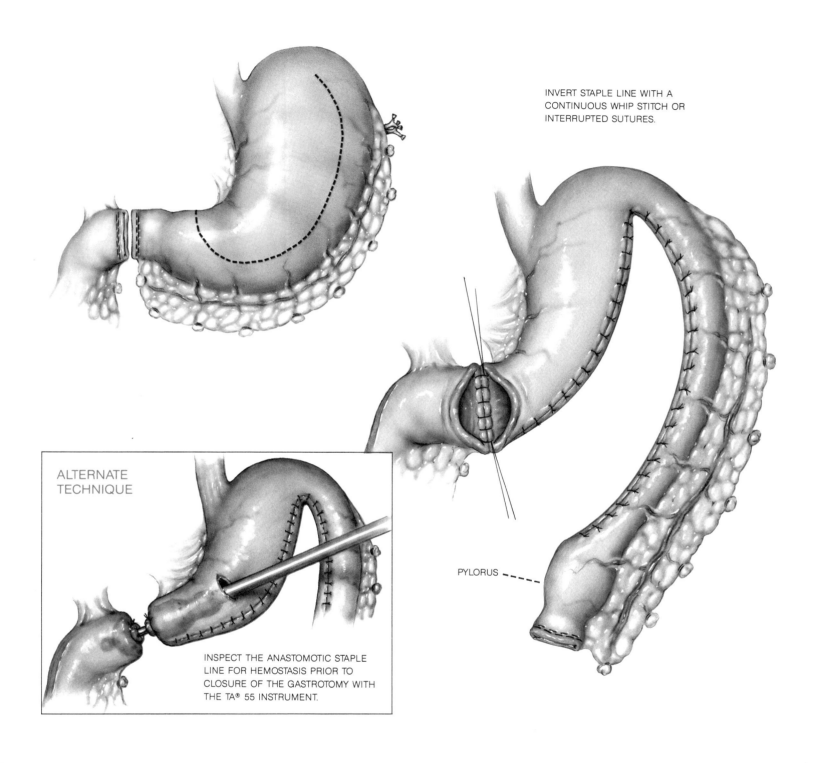

INVERT STAPLE LINE WITH A
CONTINUOUS WHIP STITCH OR
INTERRUPTED SUTURES.

ALTERNATE
TECHNIQUE

INSPECT THE ANASTOMOTIC STAPLE
LINE FOR HEMOSTASIS PRIOR TO
CLOSURE OF THE GASTROTOMY WITH
THE TA® 55 INSTRUMENT.

PYLORUS

The added length of 6-8 cm. for high anastomosis in the neck is achieved by preserving the right side of the gastroepiploic arcade and including the pylorus and first portion of the duodenum in the construction of the tube. The duodenum is transected 4-5 cm. distal to the pylorus using the GIA™ instrument. The tube is created by repeated applications of the GIA™ instrument, beginning on the lesser curvature approximately 2 cm. proximal to the pylorus.

The gastroduodenostomy may be performed with a two layer manual closure or using the EEA™ instrument introduced through a gastrotomy. The pharyngoduodenostomy is performed manually.

The fascia and skin are closed in the usual manner with the DFS™ instrument and the PREMIUM® skin stapler.

Esophagogastrectomy and Isoperistaltic Gastric Tube

Auto Suture® Instruments Used in an Esophagogastrectomy and Isoperistaltic Gastric Tube

See Cautions and Contraindications on page 236

INSTRUMENT	CLINICAL APPLICATION
LDS™ Instrument	Ligation and division of the omental vessels.
GIA™ Instrument	Creation of the gastric tube. Alternate technique: Anastomosis of the esophagus to the gastric tube.
EEA™ Instrument or PREMIUM CEEA™ Instrument	Anastomosis of the esophagus to the gastric tube. Alternate technique: Creation of the gastric window.
TA® 55 Instrument	Closure of the gastrotomy. Closure of the pyloroplasty incision. Alternate technique: Closure of the esophagus and the gastric stab wound.
DFS™ Instrument and PREMIUM® Skin Stapler	Closure of fascia and skin.

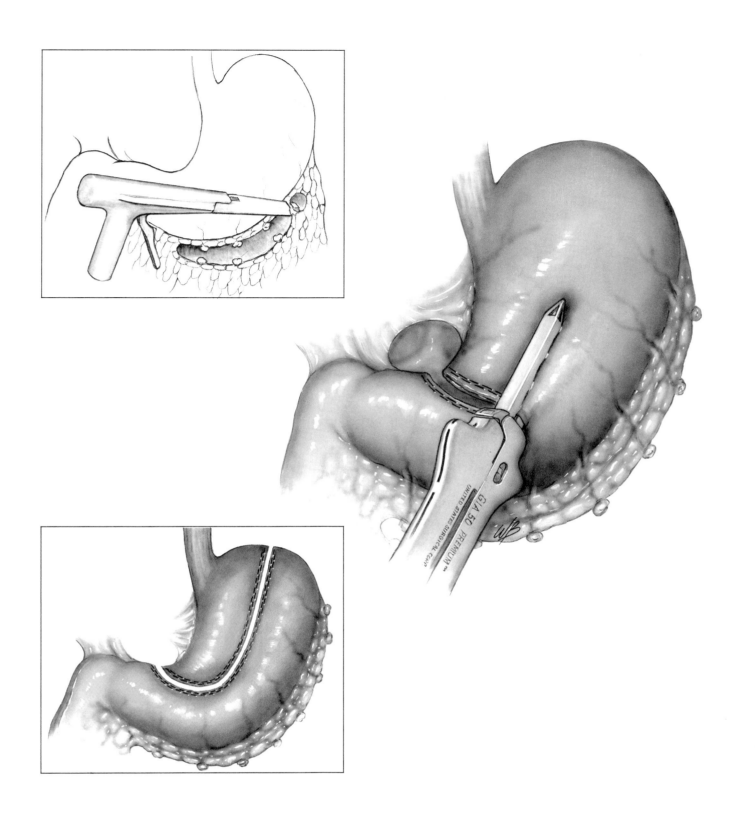

The greater curvature of the stomach is mobilized using the LDS™ instrument to ligate and divide the gastrocolic omentum peripheral to the gastroepiploic vessels.

The stomach is transected longitudinally using serial applications of the GIA™ instrument from the lower, lesser curvature to the paraesophageal gastric fundus. In this procedure, it is recommended that the staple line be oversewn with a continuous whip stitch or interrupted sutures.

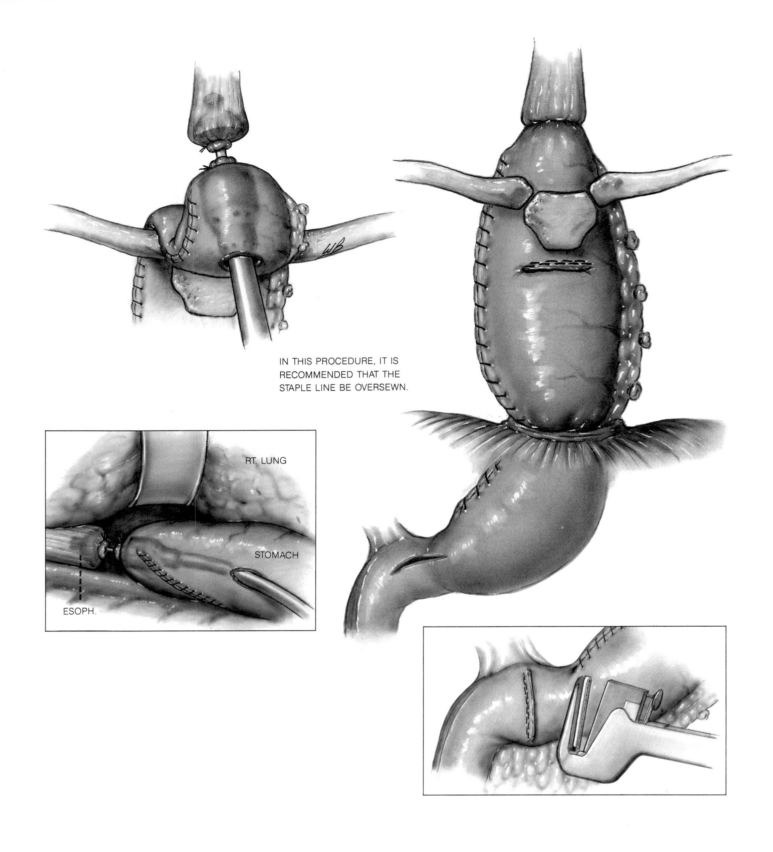

IN THIS PROCEDURE, IT IS RECOMMENDED THAT THE STAPLE LINE BE OVERSEWN.

RT. LUNG

STOMACH

ESOPH.

The long gastric tube extends with ease to the base of the neck or the apex of the right chest cavity. The esophagogastrostomy may be performed above or just below the clavicles using the EEA™ instrument introduced through a gastrotomy. Inspect the anastomosis for hemostasis prior to closure of the gastrotomy with the TA® 55 instrument.

A Heineke-Mikulicz pyloroplasty is also performed. With this technique, a smaller segment of stomach is resected than in esophagogastrectomy with a short greater curvature tube. This procedure is often preferred for carcinoma of the lower third of the esophagus.

Alternate Technique of Anastomosis

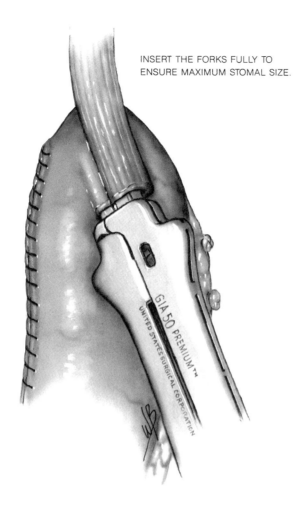

INSERT THE FORKS FULLY TO
ENSURE MAXIMUM STOMAL SIZE.

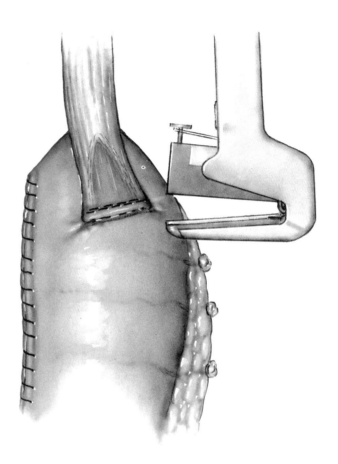

CARE MUST BE TAKEN TO
OVERLAP THE ENDS OF THE
PREVIOUS STAPLE LINES.

The esophagogastrostomy may be performed using the GIA™ instrument. A 1 cm. stab wound is made in the proximal gastric tube. Insert one fork of the instrument into the gastric tube and one fork into the esophagus. Close the instrument and fire the staples. Inspect the anastomosis for hemostasis prior to closure of the common opening with the TA® 55 instrument.

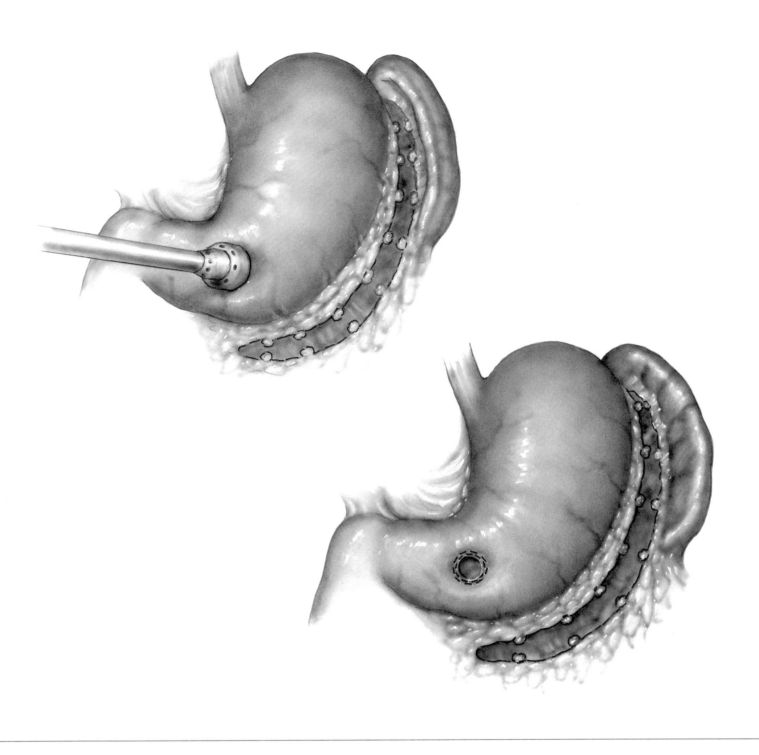

The greater curvature of the stomach is mobilized using the LDS™ instrument to ligate and divide the omentum peripheral to the gastroepiploic vessels and preserving the spleen.

The EEA™ instrument is used to create a window in the antrum of the stomach approximately 4-5 cm. proximal to the pylorus and 3 cm. from the greater curvature.

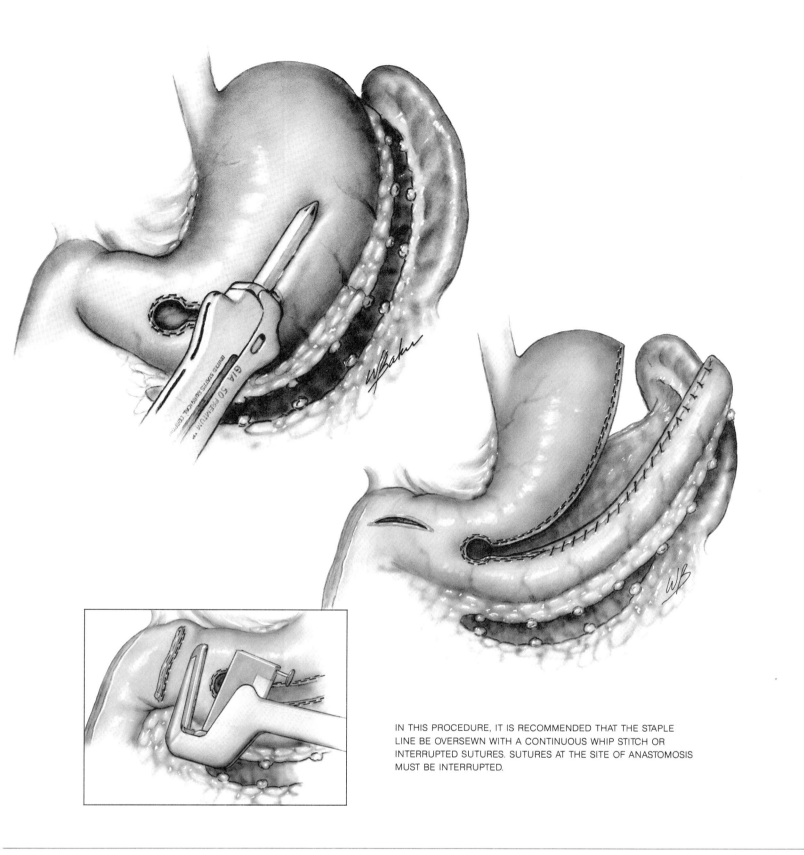

IN THIS PROCEDURE, IT IS RECOMMENDED THAT THE STAPLE
LINE BE OVERSEWN WITH A CONTINUOUS WHIP STITCH OR
INTERRUPTED SUTURES. SUTURES AT THE SITE OF ANASTOMOSIS
MUST BE INTERRUPTED.

The gastric tube is created by serial applications of
the GIA™ instrument. The first application of the instrument is made through the window and parallel to the
greater curvature of the stomach. Reapplications are
continued proximally to the lateral apex of the fundus.
A Kocher maneuver is performed to free the gastric
tube to reach the desired height.

A Heineke-Mikulicz pyloroplasty and esophagogastrostomy are performed.

This procedure is often preferred in esophageal
replacement for benign lesions or for palliative
bypass of inoperable malignant lesions where
continued esophagogastric drainage is important.

Short Isoperistaltic Gastric Tube

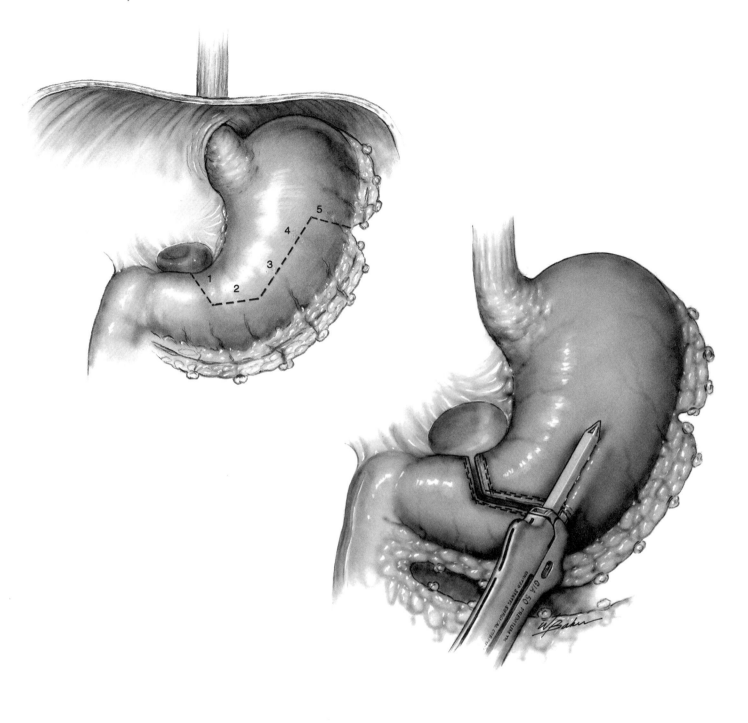

The stomach is mobilized using the LDS™ instrument to ligate and divide the omental vessels as shown. The gastroepiploic arcade is left intact to preserve the vascular supply to the gastric tube.

The proximal gastrectomy and distal gastric tube construction are performed by serial applications of the GIA™ instrument. The tube is created from the lesser curvature of the stomach to the greater curvature with five applications of the instrument as illustrated.

A Kocher maneuver is performed to free the gastric tube to reach the desired height.

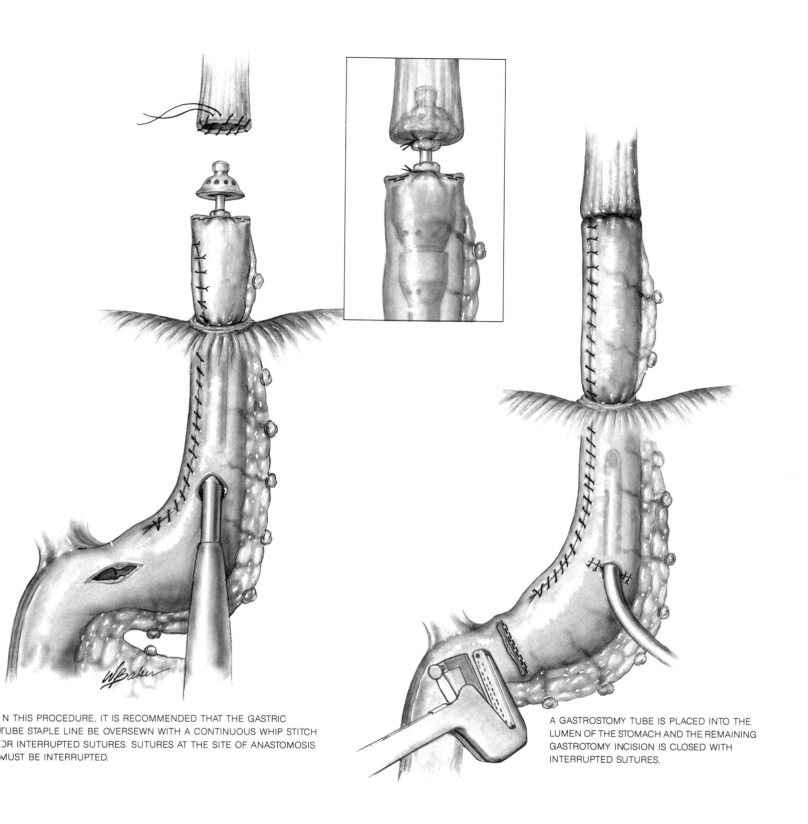

IN THIS PROCEDURE, IT IS RECOMMENDED THAT THE GASTRIC TUBE STAPLE LINE BE OVERSEWN WITH A CONTINUOUS WHIP STITCH OR INTERRUPTED SUTURES. SUTURES AT THE SITE OF ANASTOMOSIS MUST BE INTERRUPTED.

A GASTROSTOMY TUBE IS PLACED INTO THE LUMEN OF THE STOMACH AND THE REMAINING GASTROTOMY INCISION IS CLOSED WITH INTERRUPTED SUTURES.

The esophagus is transected completing the resection and the proximal esophagus is prepared with a purse string suture.

An incision is made at the center of the transverse staple line closure on the proximal end of the gastric tube and a manual purse string suture is placed. The EEA™ instrument, without anvil, is introduced through a low gastrotomy. Advance the center rod through the gastric tube opening and tie the purse string suture. Place the anvil on the center rod.

Introduce the anvil into the esophagus and tie the purse string suture. Close the EEA™ instrument and fire the staples. Remove the instrument and inspect the anastomotic staple line for hemostasis.

A Heineke-Mikulicz pyloroplasty is performed.

This procedure is often used for carcinoma at the esophagogastric junction.

The fascia and skin are closed in the usual manner with the DFS™ instrument and the PREMIUM® skin stapler.

Esophagogastrectomy and Colon Replacement

Auto Suture® Instruments Used in an Esophagogastrectomy and Colon Replacement

See Cautions and Contraindications on page 236

INSTRUMENT	CLINICAL APPLICATION
LDS™ Instrument	Ligation and division of the mesenteric vessels.
TA® 30 Instrument	Closure of the base of the appendix.
GIA™ Instrument	Closure and transection of the terminal ileum and transverse colon. Anastomosis of the ileum and transverse colon. Anastomosis of the stomach to the colon segment. Anastomosis of the esophagus to the colon segment. Anastomosis of the antrum of the stomach and the duodenum.
TA® 90 Instrument	Closure of the gastric fundus.
TA® 55 Instrument	Closure of the intestinal stab wounds. Closure of the gastric and colonic stab wounds. Closure of the esophagus and the colonic stab wound. Closure of the pyloroplasty incision.
DFS™ Instrument and PREMIUM® Skin Stapler	Closure of fascia and skin.

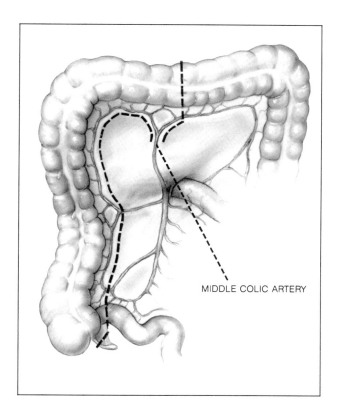

MIDDLE COLIC ARTERY

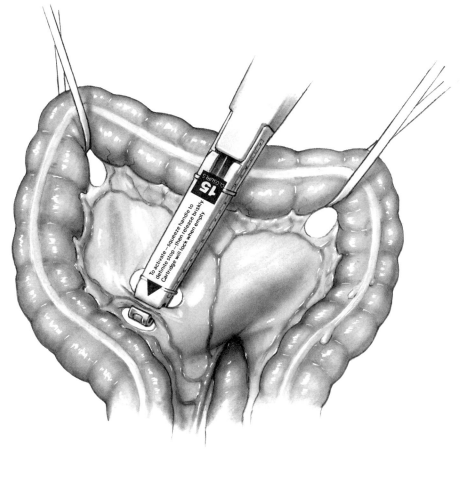

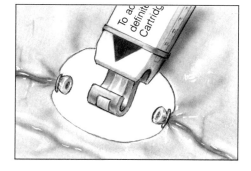

Although selection of a suitable segment of bowel for esophageal replacement varies, the procedure is illustrated using the right colon.

The right colon is mobilized using the LDS™ instrument to ligate and divide the right colic and ileocolic vessels, preserving the middle colic artery and vein and the marginal artery.

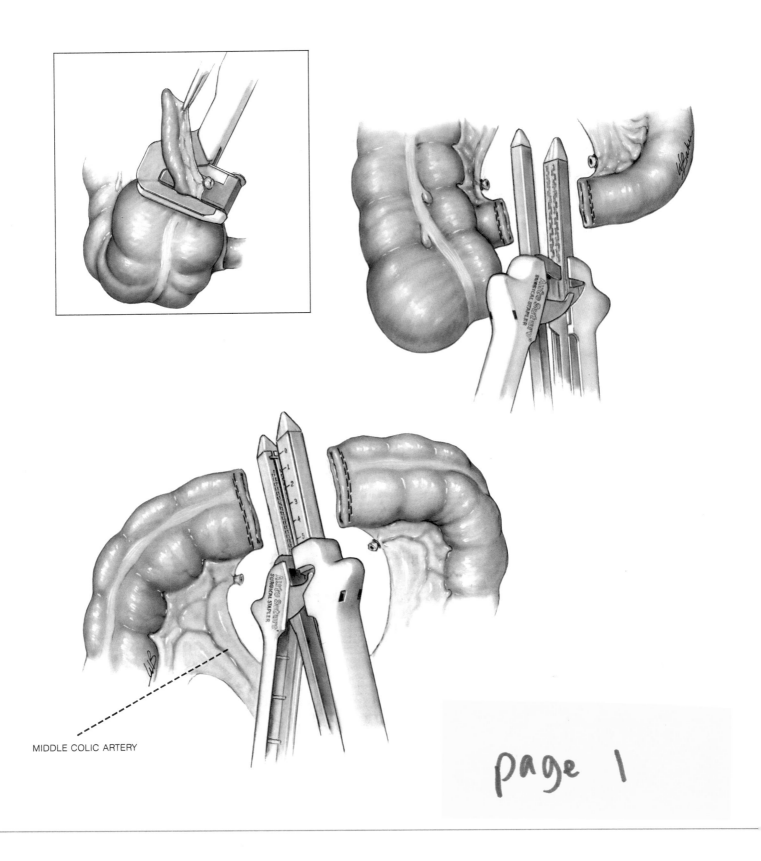

MIDDLE COLIC ARTERY

page 1

The mesoappendix is ligated and divided using the LDS™ instrument and an incidental appendectomy is performed using the TA® 30 instrument.

The right colon is isolated with two applications of the GIA™ instrument. Place the instrument around the terminal ileum in a scissor-like fashion, close the instrument and fire the staples. Two double staggered rows of staples seal the ileum; simultaneously, the knife blade in the instrument transects the bowel between the two double staple lines. A second application of the GIA™ instrument on the transverse colon completes the isolation of the right colon.

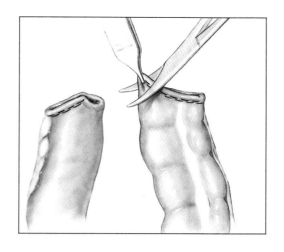

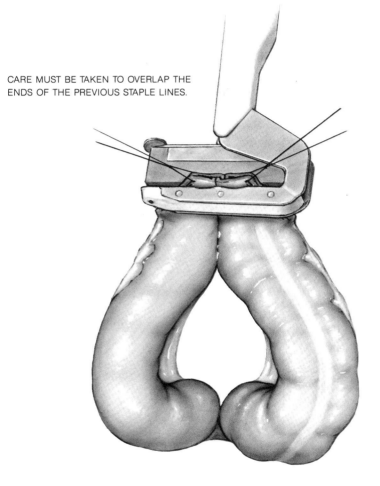

CARE MUST BE TAKEN TO OVERLAP THE
ENDS OF THE PREVIOUS STAPLE LINES.

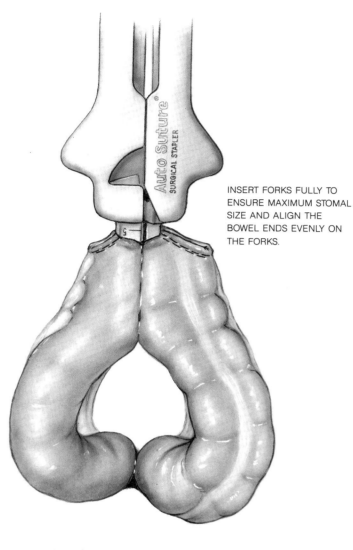

INSERT FORKS FULLY TO
ENSURE MAXIMUM STOMAL
SIZE AND ALIGN THE
BOWEL ENDS EVENLY ON
THE FORKS.

ALWAYS INSPECT THE ANASTOMOTIC
STAPLE LINES FOR HEMOSTASIS PRIOR
TO CLOSURE OF THE STAB WOUND.

page 2

Intestinal continuity is re-established by performing a functional end-to-end anastomosis. Excise the antimesenteric corners of the staple line closure of both the ileum and transverse colon, approximate the bowel loops and insert one fork of the GIA™ instrument into each bowel lumen. Close the instrument and fire the staples. The bowel walls are joined with two double staggered staple lines; simultaneously, the knife blade in the instrument divides between the two double staple lines creating a stoma. Close the now common opening with the TA® 55 instrument.

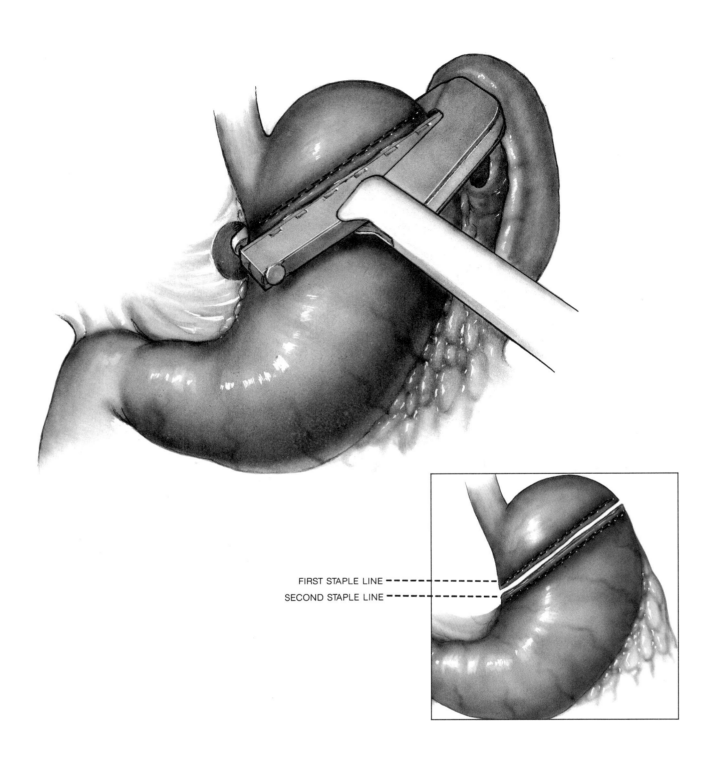

FIRST STAPLE LINE
SECOND STAPLE LINE

The gastric fundus is stapled with two applications of the TA® 90 instrument. Following the first application, the TA® 90 instrument is reapplied parallel and distal to the previous staple line. After the second application of the instrument, the stomach is transected between the two double staple lines using the superior edge of the instrument as a cutting guide. Both the gastric pouch and the specimen side remain closed, which reduces intraperitoneal soilage.

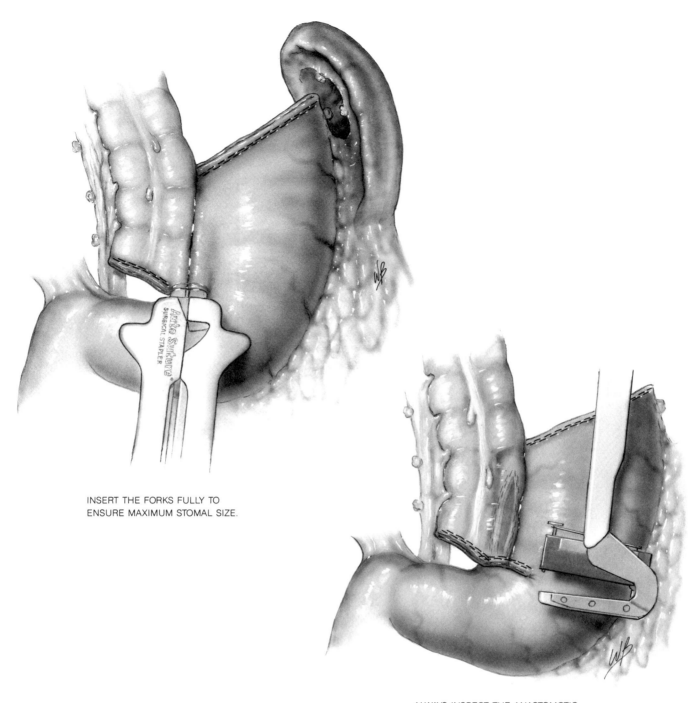

INSERT THE FORKS FULLY TO
ENSURE MAXIMUM STOMAL SIZE.

ALWAYS INSPECT THE ANASTOMOTIC
STAPLE LINE FOR HEMOSTASIS BEFORE
CLOSING THE NOW COMMON OPENING.

The isolated colon with its middle colic pedicle is then passed posterior to the stomach. The anti-mesenteric corner of the distal colonic staple line is excised, a stab wound is made into the anterior mid-gastric wall, and the cologastrostomy is performed with the GIA™ instrument. The common opening is closed with the TA® 55 instrument.

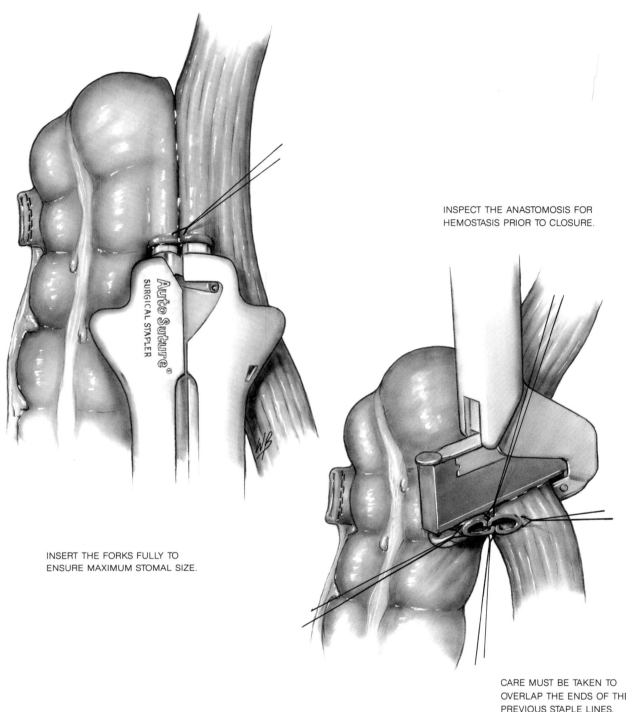

INSPECT THE ANASTOMOSIS FOR
HEMOSTASIS PRIOR TO CLOSURE.

INSERT THE FORKS FULLY TO
ENSURE MAXIMUM STOMAL SIZE.

CARE MUST BE TAKEN TO
OVERLAP THE ENDS OF THE
PREVIOUS STAPLE LINES.

The colon segment is delivered cephalad through a retrosternal tunnel and the esophagocolostomy is performed through a cervical incision. Make a stab wound approximately 5 cm. from the colon cul-de-sac and a corresponding stab wound in the esophagus. Insert the forks of the GIA™ instrument, close the instrument and fire the staples.

Closure of the esophagus and the colonic stab wound is performed in a single stage with one application of the TA® 55 instrument. Approximate the tissue edges with traction sutures. Incorporate the esophagus and the edges of the colonic stab wound within the instrument jaws. Apply the instrument obliquely to prevent pouching, and fire the staples. Prior to removal, use the instrument edge as a guide to excise the esophageal segment and colonic stab wound tissue protruding through the jaws.

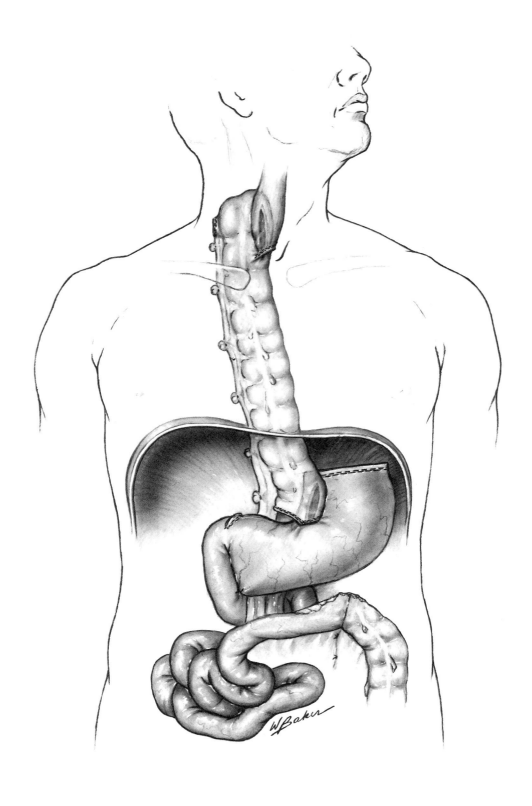

A pyloroplasty is also performed. The completed reconstruction is illustrated.

The fascia and skin are closed in the usual manner with the DFS™ instrument and the PREMIUM® skin stapler.

Palliative Side-to-Side Esophagogastrostomy

Auto Suture® Instruments Used in a Palliative Side-to-Side Esophagogastrostomy

See Cautions and Contraindications on page 236

INSTRUMENT	CLINICAL APPLICATION
LDS™ Instrument	Ligation and division of the vasa brevia.
GIA™ Instrument	Anastomosis of the esophagus to the stomach.
TA® 55 Instrument	Closure of the common stab wound.
PREMIUM® Skin Stapler	Closure of skin.

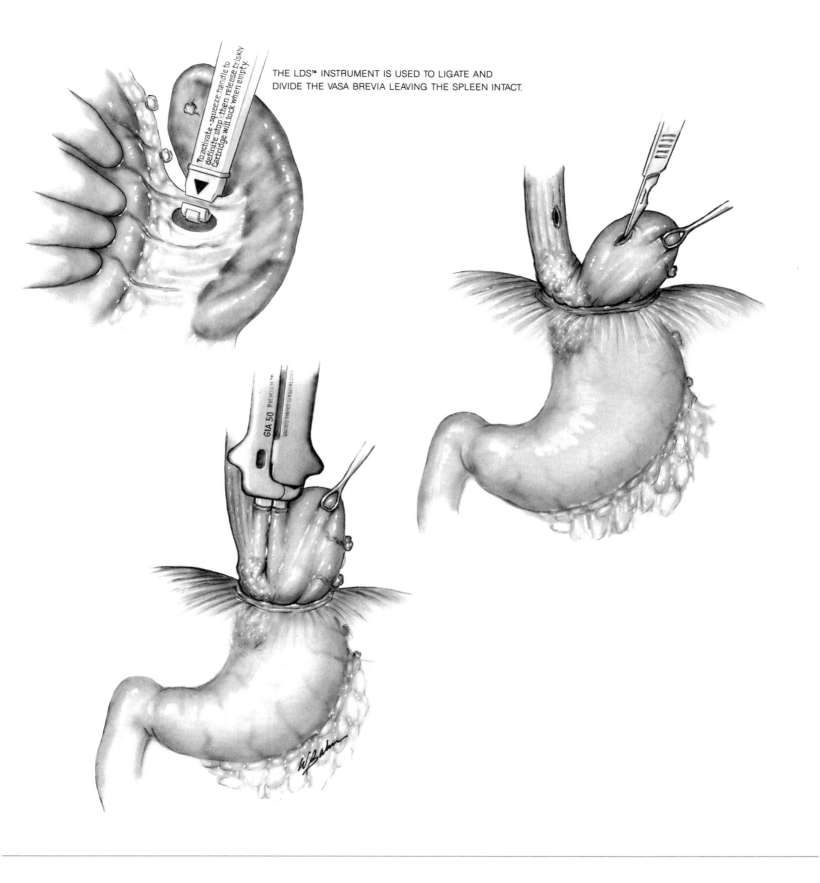

THE LDS™ INSTRUMENT IS USED TO LIGATE AND
DIVIDE THE VASA BREVIA LEAVING THE SPLEEN INTACT.

The fundus of the stomach is mobilized using the
LDS™ instrument to ligate and divide the first three or
four vasa brevia, leaving the spleen intact.

The fundus is presented into the lower mediastinum
through the enlarged diaphragmatic hiatus. The GIA™
instrument is used to perform the esophagogastrostomy.
A 1 cm. stab wound is made into the lateral wall of
the esophagus 5-6 cm. proximal to the tumor and a

corresponding stab wound is made into the medial
wall of the gastric fundus. Insert the forks of the GIA™
instrument. Close the instrument and fire the staples.
Inspect the anastomotic staple lines for hemostasis
prior to closure of the now common stab wound with
the TA® 55 instrument or with manual sutures.

The skin is closed in the usual manner with the
PREMIUM® skin stapler.

Collis-Nissen Procedure

Auto Suture® Instruments Used in a Collis-Nissen Gastroplasty and Fundoplication

See Cautions and Contraindications on page 236

INSTRUMENT	CLINICAL APPLICATION
LDS™ Instrument	Ligation and division of the vasa brevia.
GIA™ Instrument	Creation of the Collis gastric tube.
PREMIUM CEEA™ Instrument	Creation of the gastric window in an abdominal approach.
DFS™ Instrument and PREMIUM® Skin Stapler	Closure of fascia and skin.

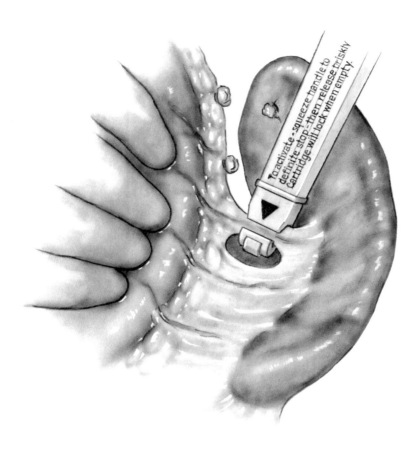

THE LDS™ INSTRUMENT IS USED TO LIGATE AND
DIVIDE THE VASA BREVIA LEAVING THE SPLEEN INTACT.

The fundus of the stomach is brought through an
enlarged diaphragmatic hiatus and mobilized using
the LDS™ instrument to ligate and divide the vasa
brevia leaving the spleen intact.

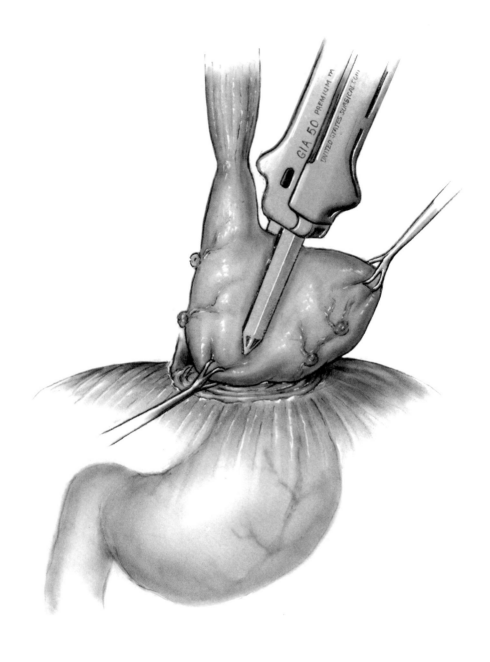

The GIA™ instrument is used to create the Collis gastric tube. Apply the GIA™ instrument across the stomach parallel to the lesser curvature and along a #50-52 F Bougie placed to dilate the stricture and calibrate the gastric tube. Close the instrument and fire the staples. The instrument places two double staggered staple lines; simultaneously, the knife blade in the instrument divides between the two double staple lines creating a 5-6 cm. gastric tube in continuity with the esophagus.

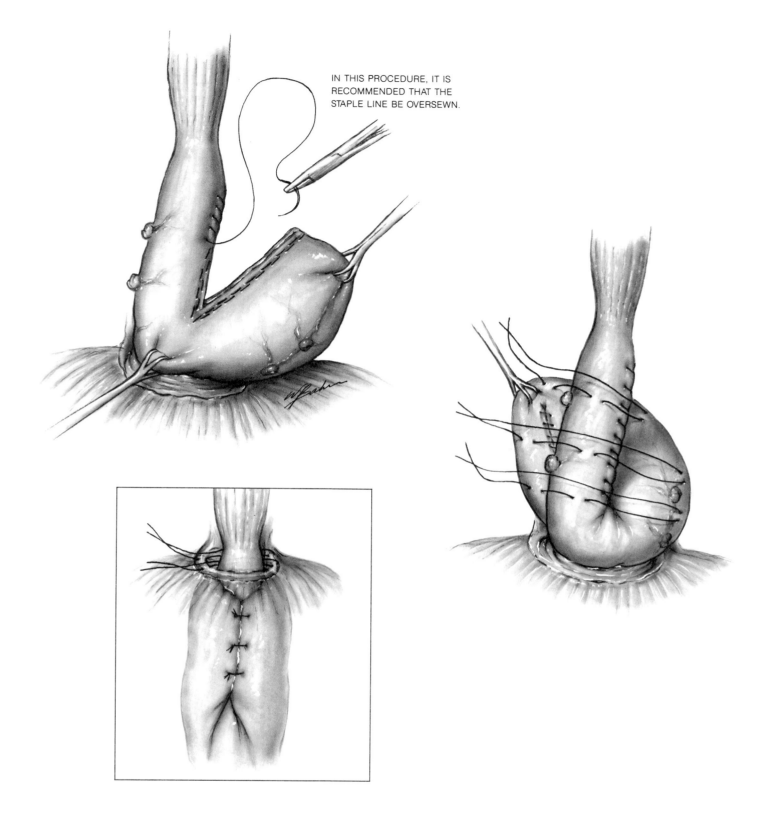

IN THIS PROCEDURE, IT IS
RECOMMENDED THAT THE
STAPLE LINE BE OVERSEWN.

In this procedure, it is recommended that the staple line be oversewn with a continuous whip stitch or interrupted sutures.

The Nissen fundoplication is performed with interrupted sutures. The stomach is replaced in the abdomen and the hiatus is sutured and closed posteriorly around the gastric tube.

Abdominal Approach

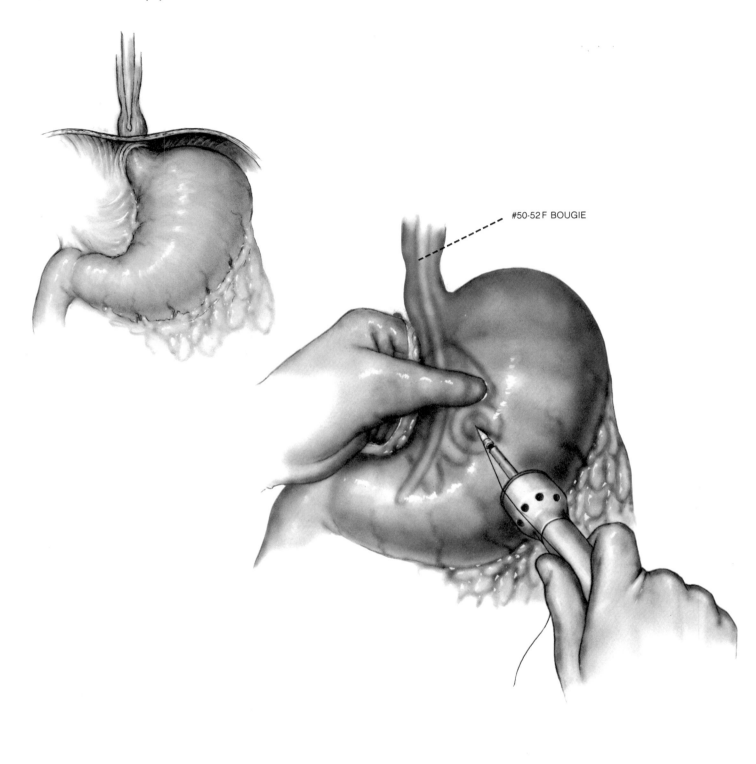

#50-52 F BOUGIE

The PREMIUM CEEA™ instrument is used to create a window through the stomach approximately 5 cm. from the esophagogastric junction and a distance equivalent to the width of the esophagus from the lesser curvature of the stomach. Make an opening in the lesser omentum and place the anvil of the

PREMIUM CEEA™ instrument against the posterior wall of the stomach at the site for the window. With the trocar tip, perforate the anterior and posterior walls of the stomach using the center of the anvil as a guide. Advance the center rod through the gastric opening.

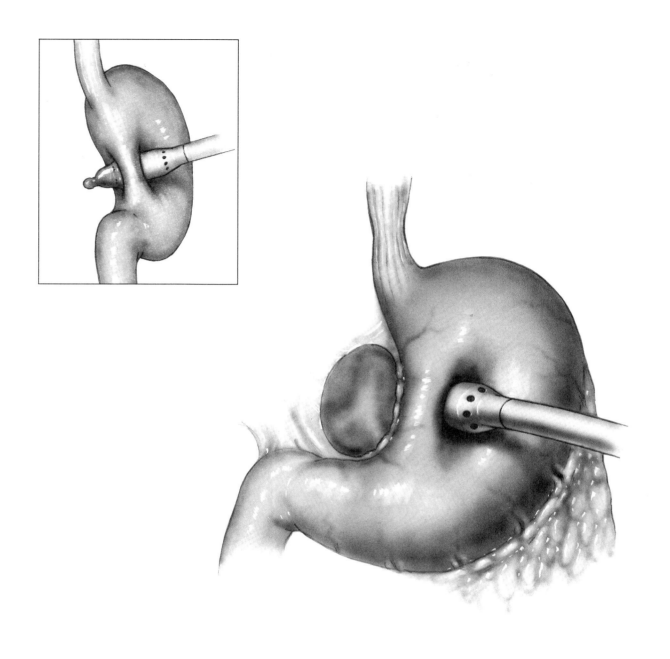

Remove the trocar tip and place the anvil on the anvil shaft. Close the instrument and fire the staples. A circular double staggered row of staples join the anterior and posterior walls of the stomach and the circular blade in the instrument cuts a window.

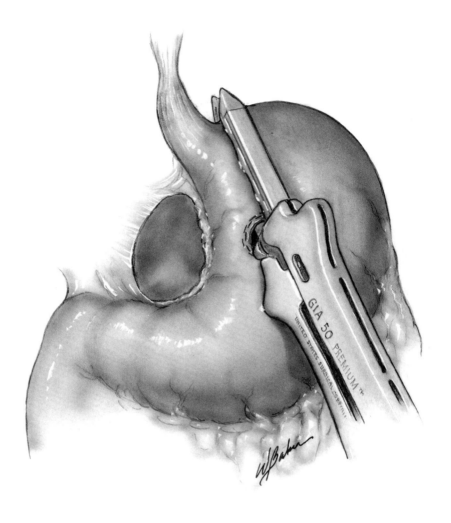

The GIA™ instrument is used to create the gastric tube. The instrument is applied through the gastric window and parallel to the lesser curvature of the stomach. In cases with a short esophagus, the GIA™ instrument may project partially into the lower mediastinum through the enlarged hiatus. The instrument is fired, creating a 5-6 cm. gastric tube in continuity with the esophagus.

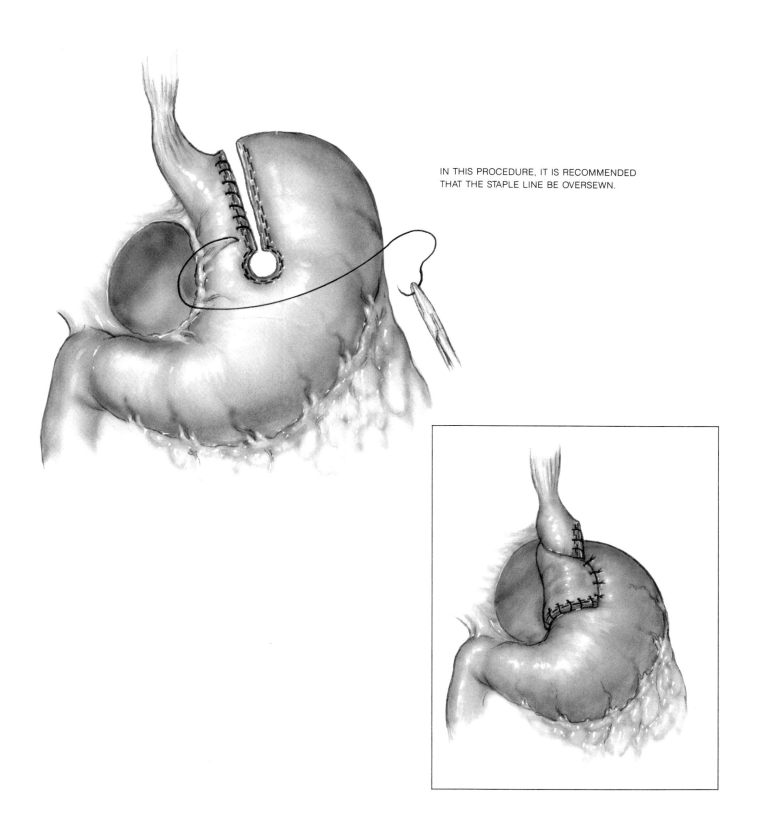

IN THIS PROCEDURE, IT IS RECOMMENDED
THAT THE STAPLE LINE BE OVERSEWN.

The fundus of the stomach is passed posteriorly around the gastric tube, through the opening in the lesser omentum and anteriorly over the gastric tube. It is sutured to the midanterior gastric wall, forming the fundoplication.

The fascia and skin are closed in the usual manner with the DFS™ instrument and the PREMIUM® skin stapler.

Zenker's Diverticulectomy

Auto Suture® Instruments Used in a
Zenker's Diverticulectomy

See Cautions and Contraindications on page 236

INSTRUMENT	CLINICAL APPLICATION
TA® 30 Instrument or TA® 55 Instrument	Closure of the base of the diverticulum.
PREMIUM® Skin Stapler	Closure of skin.

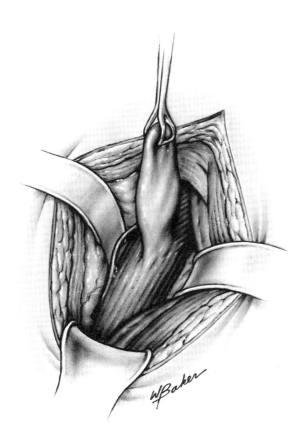

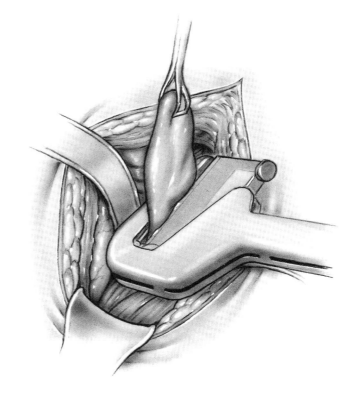

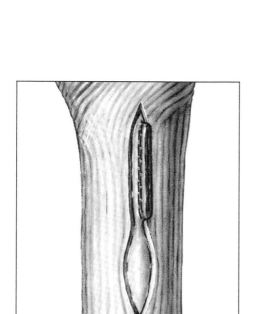

Resection of a Zenker's pharyngeal diverticulum is performed using the TA® 30 instrument or TA® 55 instrument. Following isolation of the diverticulum, it is gently elevated and the TA® 30 instrument or TA® 55 instrument is placed across the base of the diverticulum parallel to the long axis of the esophagus. Close the instrument and fire the staples.

Prior to removing the instrument, resect the diverticulum using the instrument edge as a cutting guide. No reinforcement of the staple line is required.

The usual myotomy of 2-3 cm. is performed.

The skin is closed in the usual manner with the PREMIUM® skin stapler.

Ligation of Esophageal Varices

Auto Suture® Instruments Used in Ligation of Esophageal Varices

See Cautions and Contraindications on page 236

INSTRUMENT	CLINICAL APPLICATION
GIA™ Instrument	Creation of the gastrotomy. Ligation of esophageal varices in linear staple line technique.
PREMIUM CEEA™ Instrument or EEA™ Instrument	Ligation of esophageal varices.
TA® 55 Instrument	Closure of the gastrotomy.
TA® 30 Instrument	Closure of the stab wound in linear staple line technique.
DFS™ Instrument and PREMIUM® Skin Stapler	Closure of fascia and skin.

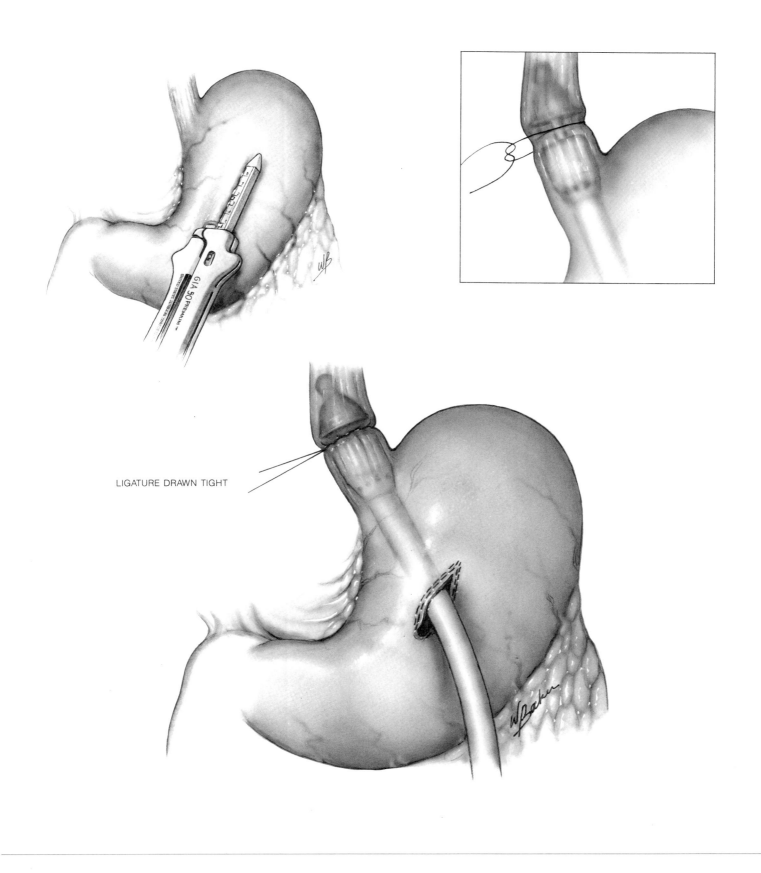

LIGATURE DRAWN TIGHT

The GIA™ instrument is used to incise the stomach and secure hemostasis of the cut edges. A 1 cm. stab wound is made into the anterior gastric wall at the level for the gastrotomy. Insert the anvil fork of the instrument into the lumen of the stomach and place the cartridge fork on the serosal surface. Close the instrument and fire the staples. Two double staggered staple lines are placed in the gastric wall and the knife blade in the instrument cuts an incision between them.

The EEA™ instrument is used for ligation of esophageal varices. Introduce the EEA™ instrument through the gastrotomy and into the distal esophagus. Open the instrument and tie a ligature around the esophagus and the center rod. Close the EEA™ instrument and fire the staples. A circular double staggered row of staples ligates the esophageal varices and the circular blade in the instrument cuts a stoma.

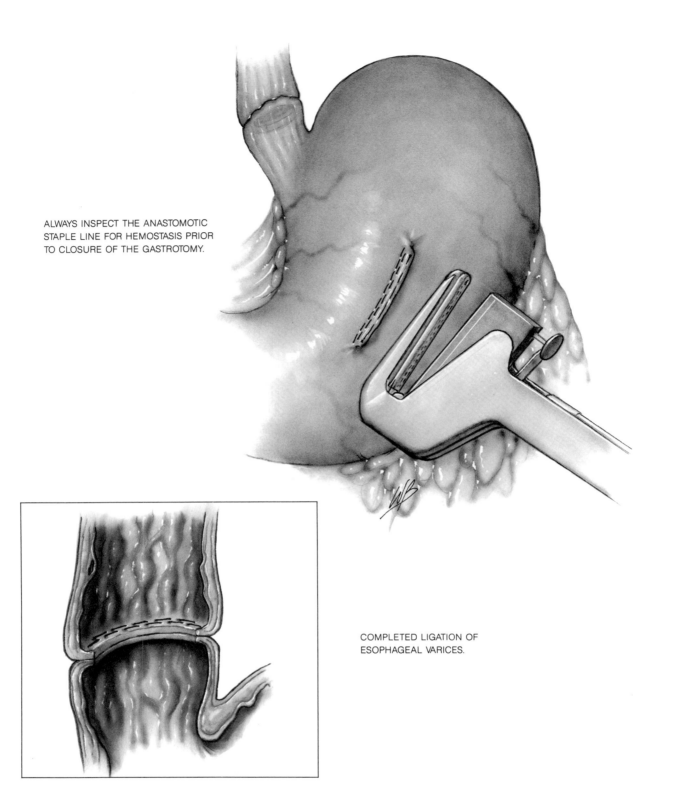

ALWAYS INSPECT THE ANASTOMOTIC
STAPLE LINE FOR HEMOSTASIS PRIOR
TO CLOSURE OF THE GASTROTOMY.

COMPLETED LIGATION OF
ESOPHAGEAL VARICES.

Open the instrument slightly and place a traction or figure-of-eight suture around the staple line. Lift the staple line over the anvil; simultaneously, gently rotate and remove the instrument.

Inspect the staple line for hemostasis prior to closing the gastrotomy with the TA® 55 instrument. Approximate the stapled edges of the gastric wall with Allis clamps or traction sutures. Slip the jaws of the TA® 55 instrument around the tissue, close the instrument and fire the staples. Before releasing the tissue, use the instrument edge as a guide to excise the margin of tissue protruding through the jaws.

Ligation of Esophageal Varices with Linear Staple Line

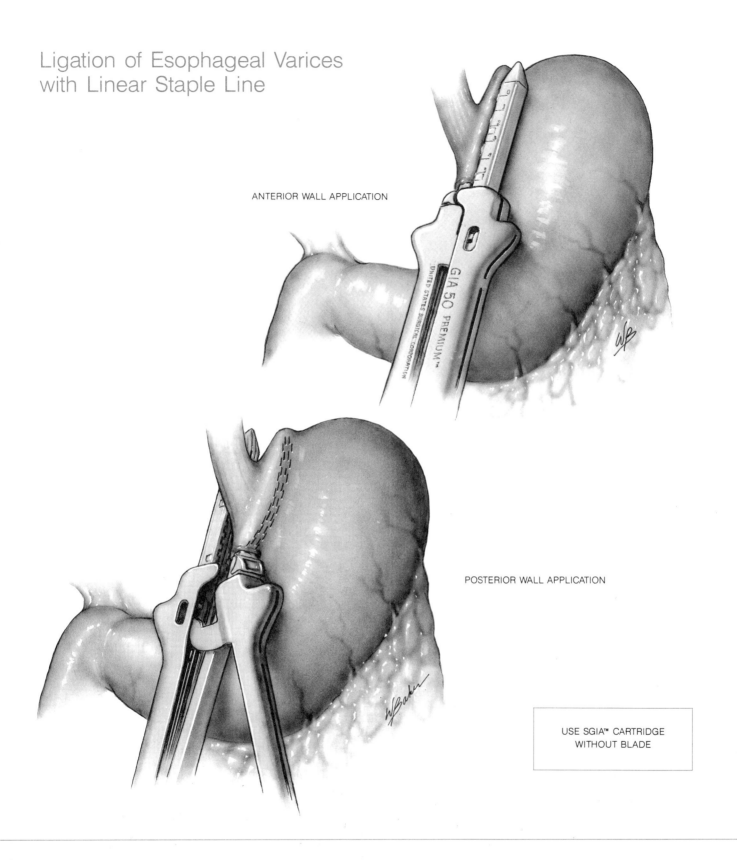

ANTERIOR WALL APPLICATION

POSTERIOR WALL APPLICATION

USE SGIA™ CARTRIDGE
WITHOUT BLADE

The esophageal varices are ligated using the GIA™ instrument with the SGIA™ disposable loading unit which contains <u>no knife</u> in the push-bar assembly. A stab wound is made on the lesser curvature, distal to the esophagogastric junction. Insert the anvil fork into the lumen of the stomach and place the cartridge fork on the anterior serosal surface. Close the instrument and fire the staples. Four parallel rows of staples ligate the varices anteriorly. The GIA™ instrument is reapplied posteriorly to complete the ligation.

The TA® 30 instrument is used to close the stab wound.

The fascia and skin are closed in the usual manner with the DFS™ instrument and the PREMIUM® skin stapler.

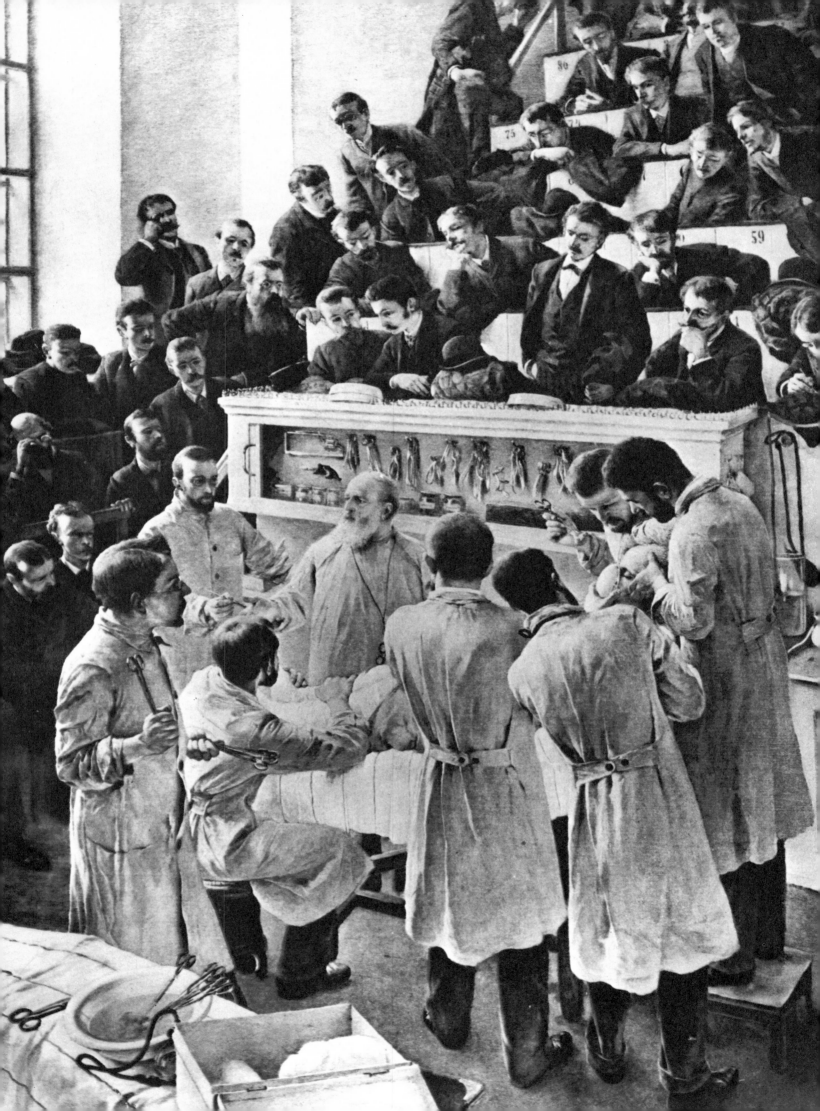

GASTRIC SURGERY

Theodore Billroth lecturing at Vienna General Hospital.
(From a painting by A.F. Seligman, 1880)

55

Billroth II

Auto Suture® Instruments Used in a
Billroth II Procedure

See Cautions and Contraindications on page 236

INSTRUMENT	CLINICAL APPLICATION
LDS™ Instrument	Ligation and division of the omental vessels.
TA® 55 Instrument	Closure of the duodenum. Closure of the gastrojejunal stab wound. Closure of the jejunojejunal stab wound for the Roux-en-Y. Alternate technique: Closure of the gastrotomy.
TA® 90 Instrument	Closure of the gastric pouch.
GIA™ Instrument	Anastomosis of the jejunum to the gastric pouch. Closure and transection of the jejunum and anastomosis of the proximal and distal jejunum for the Roux-en-Y. Alternate technique: Creation of the gastrotomy.
EEA™ Instrument or PREMIUM CEEA™ Instrument	Alternate technique: Anastomosis of the jejunum to the gastric pouch.
DFS™ Instrument and PREMIUM® Skin Stapler	Closure of fascia and skin.

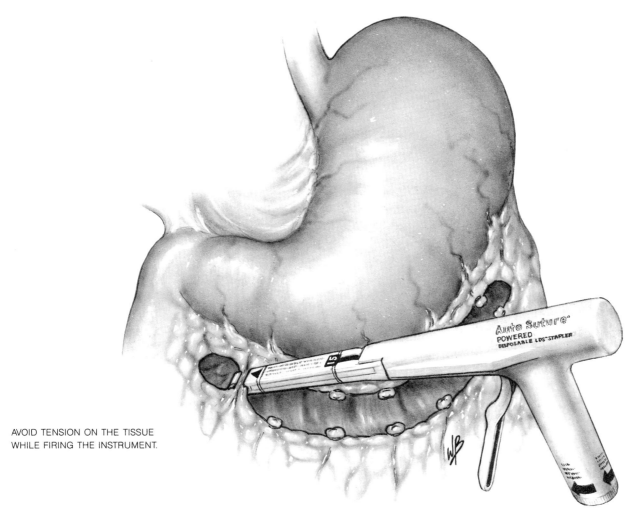

AVOID TENSION ON THE TISSUE
WHILE FIRING THE INSTRUMENT.

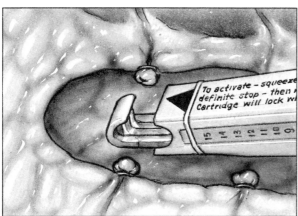

ASSURE THAT THE TISSUE AND STAPLES
ARE FREE OF THE CARTRIDGE PRIOR
TO REMOVING THE INSTRUMENT.

The stomach is mobilized using the LDS™ instrument to ligate and divide the omental vessels. Slip the tissue to be ligated into the jaw of the LDS™ instrument and fire the staples. Two staples ligate the vessel and a knife blade divides the vessel between the staples.

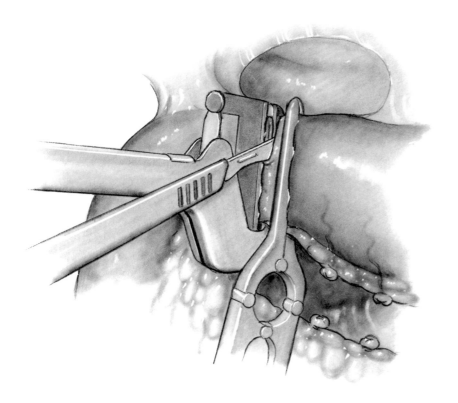

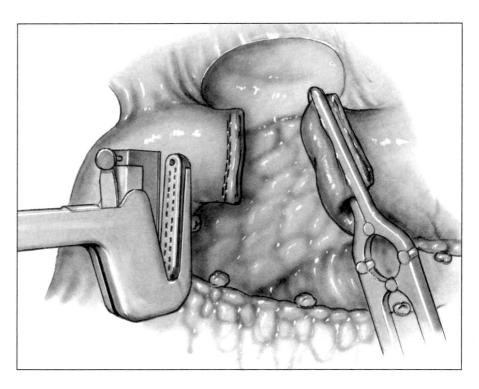

The TA® 55 instrument is used to close the duodenum. Slip the jaws of the instrument around the duodenum at the point of transection, close the instrument and fire the staples. Prior to removing the instrument, place a clamp on the specimen side and use the TA® 55 instrument edge as a cutting guide to transect the duodenum.

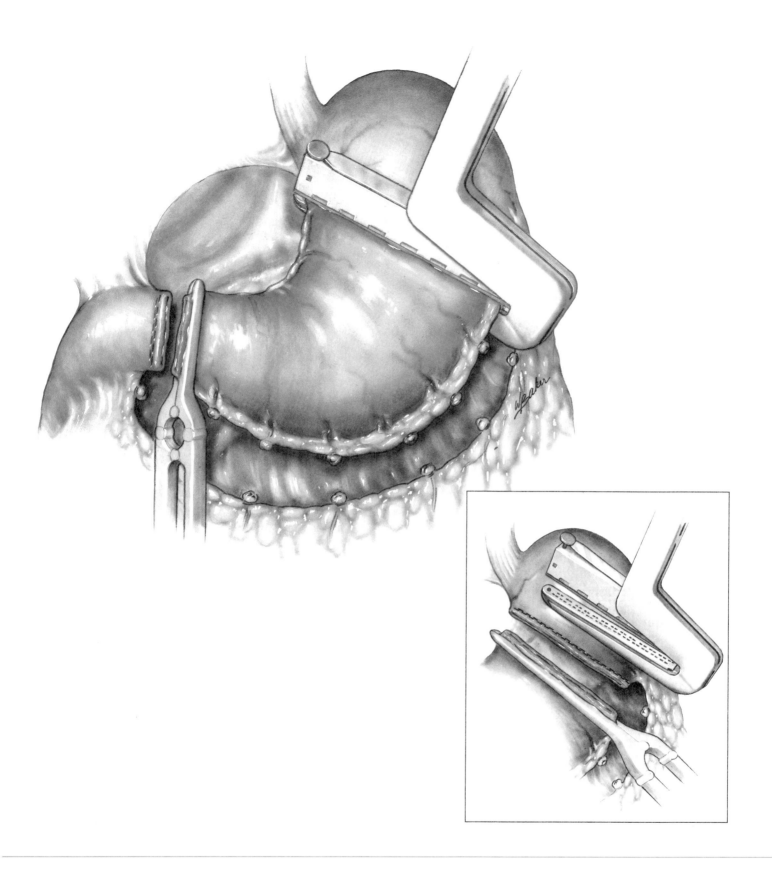

The TA® 90 instrument is used to close the gastric pouch. Slip the jaws of the instrument around the stomach at the level of transection. Close the instrument and fire the staples. Before removing the instrument, place a clamp on the specimen side and transect the stomach using the TA® 90 instrument edge as a cutting guide. There may be some oozing along the gastric staple line which usually stops spontaneously. Occasionally a bleeder along the cut edge occurs and should be ligated manually.

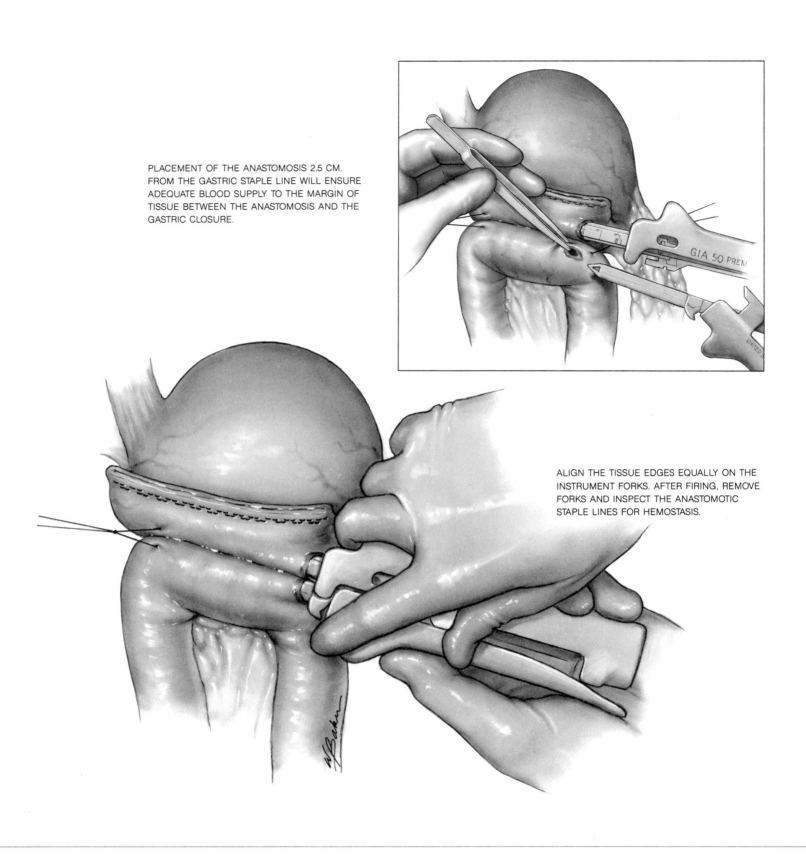

PLACEMENT OF THE ANASTOMOSIS 2.5 CM.
FROM THE GASTRIC STAPLE LINE WILL ENSURE
ADEQUATE BLOOD SUPPLY TO THE MARGIN OF
TISSUE BETWEEN THE ANASTOMOSIS AND THE
GASTRIC CLOSURE.

ALIGN THE TISSUE EDGES EQUALLY ON THE
INSTRUMENT FORKS. AFTER FIRING, REMOVE
FORKS AND INSPECT THE ANASTOMOTIC
STAPLE LINES FOR HEMOSTASIS.

The gastrojejunostomy is performed with the GIA™ instrument. With the aid of traction sutures, approximate the antimesenteric border of the jejunum to the stomach 2.5 cm. from the gastric staple line. Make a 1 cm. stab wound into the lumen of the stomach 2.5 cm. from the greater curvature, and a corresponding stab wound into the lumen of the jejunum. Insert the cartridge fork of the instrument into the lumen of the stomach and the anvil fork into the lumen of the jejunum. Insert the forks of the GIA™ instrument fully to obtain maximum stomal size. Close the instrument and fire the staples. Two double staggered rows of staples join the organs; simultaneously, the knife blade in the instrument cuts between the two double staple lines creating a stoma. To avoid enlarging the now common stab wound, open the GIA™ instrument handle slightly to free the tissue from the forks and slide the instrument out.

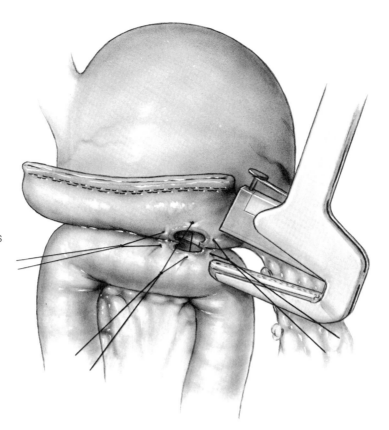

ENSURE THAT ALL TISSUE LAYERS AND
THE END STAPLES OF THE ANASTOMOSIS
ARE INCORPORATED WITHIN THE JAWS.

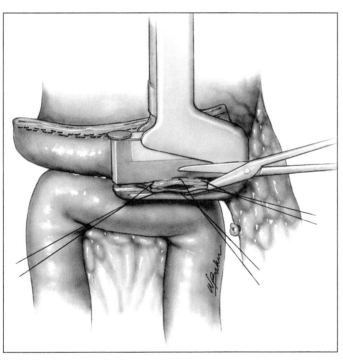

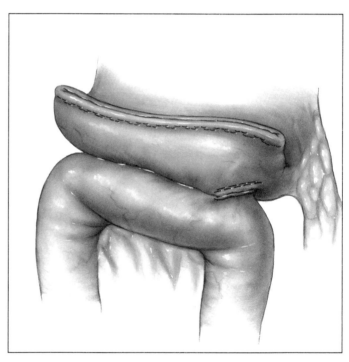

Always inspect the anastomotic staple lines for
hemostasis before closing the now common stab
wound with the TA® 55 instrument. Place an everting
traction suture around each anastomotic staple line
and distract the sutures. Place a third traction suture
or Allis clamp at the midpoint of the stab wound to
approximate the tissue edges. The wound edges are
approximated in an everted manner, with the

anastomotic staple lines held in opposition and the
stoma held open. Slip the jaws of the TA® 55
instrument around the tissue beneath the traction
sutures. Close the instrument and fire the staples. Prior
to releasing the tissue, use the instrument edge as a
guide to excise the margin of tissue protruding
through the jaws.

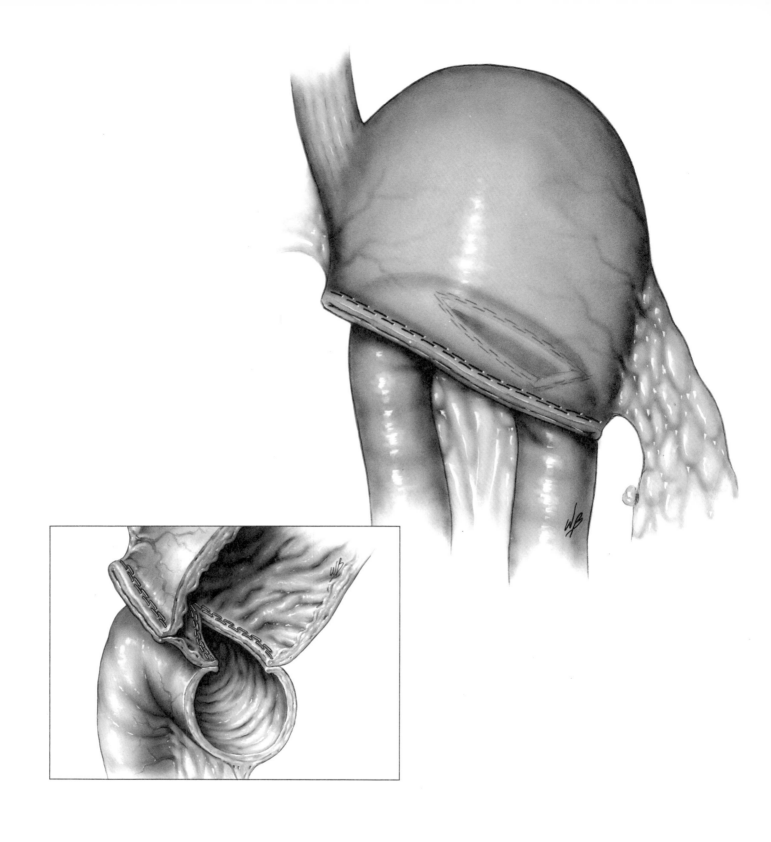

The resulting anastomosis is illustrated with the
anterior gastric wall made transparent to depict the
reconstruction.

Alternate Approaches

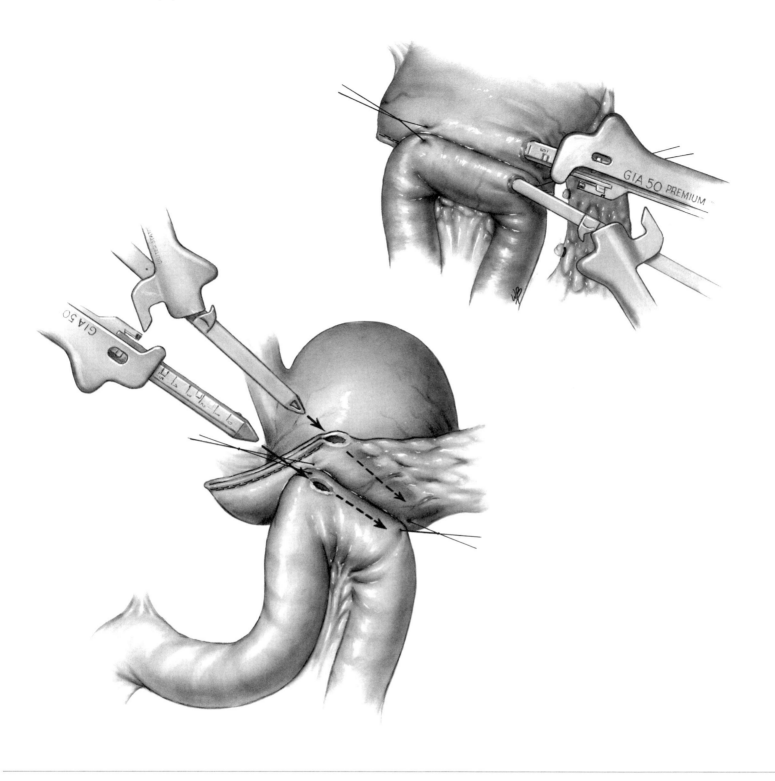

The gastrojejunostomy may be performed on the anterior gastric wall or by excising a corner of the gastric staple line and applying the GIA™ instrument along the posterior gastric wall, parallel to the greater curvature.

Anastomosis Followed By Resection

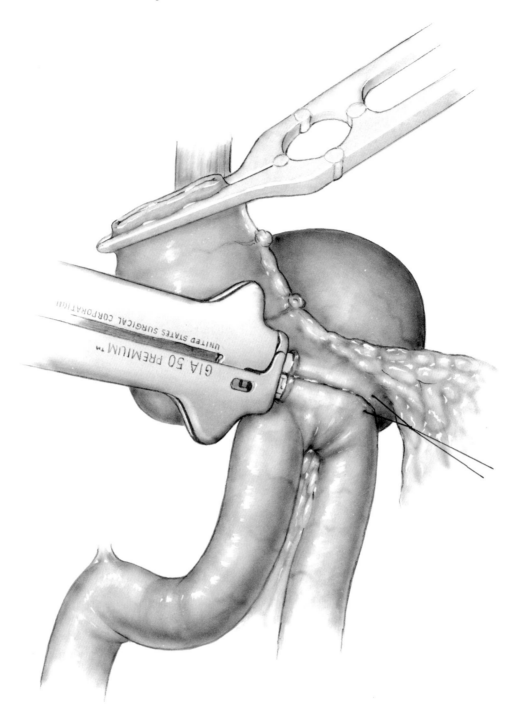

The GIA™ instrument is used to perform the anastomosis. Using the gastric specimen for traction, make a 1 cm. stab wound into the posterior wall of the stomach at the site of the planned anastomosis and a corresponding stab wound into the antimesenteric border of the jejunum. Insert the forks of the GIA™ instrument, close the instrument and fire the staples. Remove the instrument and inspect the anastomotic staple lines for hemostasis.

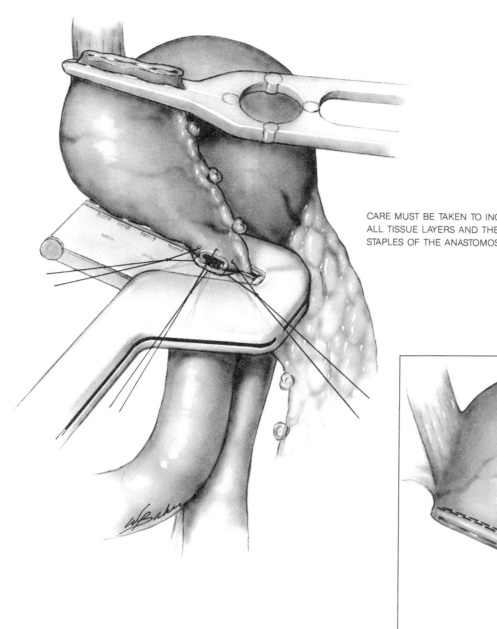

CARE MUST BE TAKEN TO INCORPORATE
ALL TISSUE LAYERS AND THE END
STAPLES OF THE ANASTOMOSIS.

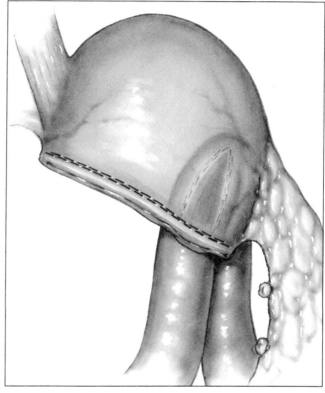

Place an everting traction suture around each anastomotic staple line and hold the staple lines in opposition. To simultaneously close the now common stab wound and resect the specimen, place the TA® 90 instrument around the stomach at the level of transection. Care is taken to include the two lips of the common stab wound on the specimen side of the instrument. Close the instrument and fire the staples. Resect the stomach using the instrument edge as a cutting guide prior to removing the instrument.

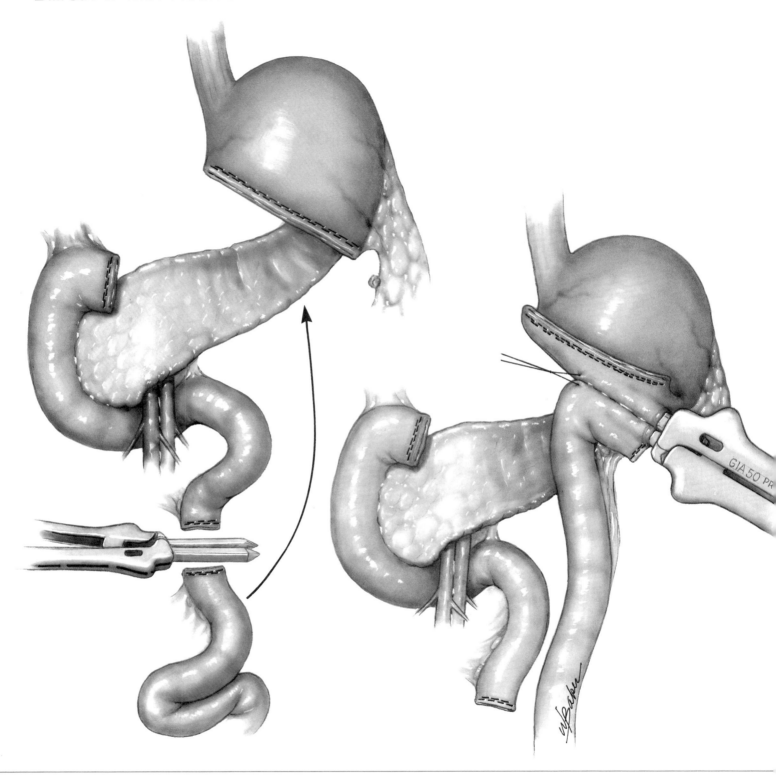

The stomach is mobilized and resected as previously described.

The GIA™ instrument is used to transect the jejunum. Place the instrument around the jejunum at the point of transection in a scissor-like fashion, close the instrument and fire the staples. Two double staggered rows of staples seal the jejunum; simultaneously, the knife blade in the instrument transects the bowel between the two double staple lines.

The gastrojejunostomy is performed with the GIA™ instrument. Approximate the antimesenteric border of the distal jejunum to the stomach 2.5 cm. from the gastric staple line. Make a 1 cm. stab wound into the lumen of the stomach 2.5 cm. from the greater curvature and excise the antimesenteric corner of the staple line closure of the jejunum. Insert the cartridge fork of the instrument into the lumen of the stomach and the anvil fork into the lumen of the jejunum. Close the instrument and fire the staples. Inspect the anastomotic staple lines for hemostasis prior to closing the now common opening with the TA® 55 instrument.

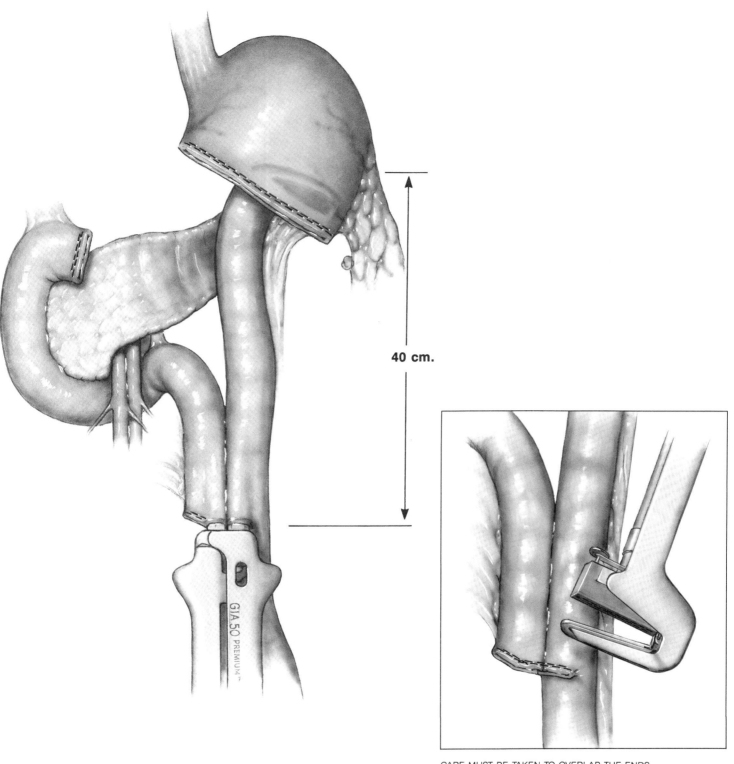

40 cm.

CARE MUST BE TAKEN TO OVERLAP THE ENDS
OF THE PREVIOUSLY PLACED STAPLE LINES.

The GIA™ instrument is used to perform the Roux-en-Y jejunojejunostomy. Make a 1 cm. stab wound into the antimesenteric border of the efferent limb of the jejunum approximately 40 cm. distal to the gastro-jejunostomy and excise the antimesenteric corner of

the staple line closure of the afferent limb. Insert one fork of the GIA™ instrument into each bowel lumen. Close the instrument and fire the staples. Inspect the anastomotic staple lines for hemostasis prior to closing the now common opening with the TA® 55 instrument.

Alternate Technique

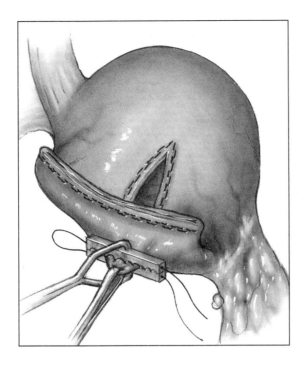

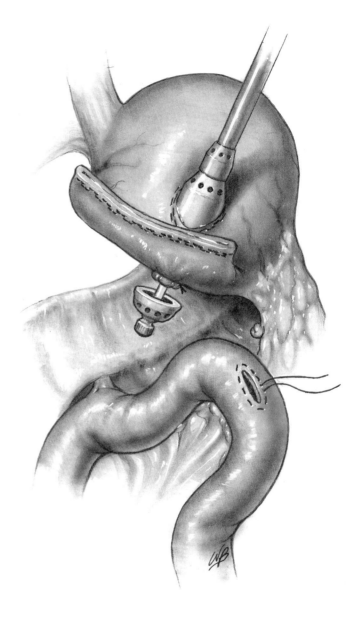

The stomach is mobilized and resected as previously described. The GIA™ instrument is used to create a gastrotomy in the anterior gastric wall.

Identify the location of the anastomosis on the posterior gastric wall 3-4 cm. proximal to the staple line closure and at least 3-4 cm. from the greater curvature of the stomach. With an Allis clamp, grasp all tissue layers of the gastric wall. Apply the purse string instrument and purse string suture. Excise the excess tissue using the purse string instrument as a cutting guide.

The EEA™ instrument is used to perform the gastrojejunostomy. Introduce the instrument, without anvil, through the gastrotomy. Remove the purse string instrument and advance the center rod of the EEA™ instrument through the posterior gastric wall. Open the instrument, tie the purse string suture and place the anvil on the center rod.

Make a 2.5-3 cm. longitudinal incision along the antimesenteric border of the jejunum at the site of the anastomosis. Place a manual purse string suture around the incision.

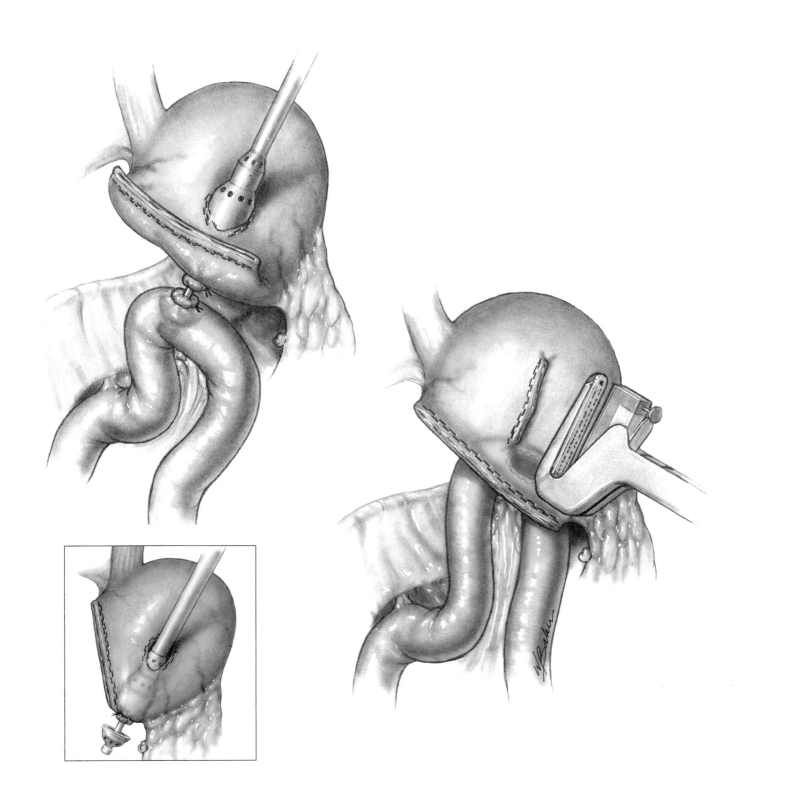

Introduce the anvil into the jejunum. The use of three Allis clamps or three traction sutures on the tissue edges may facilitate insertion of the anvil. Tie the purse string suture, close the EEA™ instrument and fire the staples. Open the instrument slightly, gently rotate and remove the instrument. Inspect the anastomotic staple line for hemostasis prior to closure of the gastrotomy with the TA® 55 instrument.

The gastrojejunostomy may be performed through the gastric staple line at the greater curvature of the stomach.

The fascia and skin are closed in the usual manner with the DFS™ instrument and the PREMIUM® skin stapler.

Billroth I

Auto Suture® Instruments Used in a Billroth I Procedure

See Cautions and Contraindications on page 236

INSTRUMENT	CLINICAL APPLICATION
LDS™ Instrument	Ligation and division of the omental vessels.
TA® 90 Instrument	Closure of the gastric pouch.
GIA™ Instrument	Creation of the gastrotomy.
EEA™ Instrument or PREMIUM CEEA™ Instrument	Anastomosis of the duodenum to the gastric pouch.
TA® 55 Instrument	Closure of the gastrotomy.
DFS™ Instrument and PREMIUM® Skin Stapler	Closure of fascia and skin.

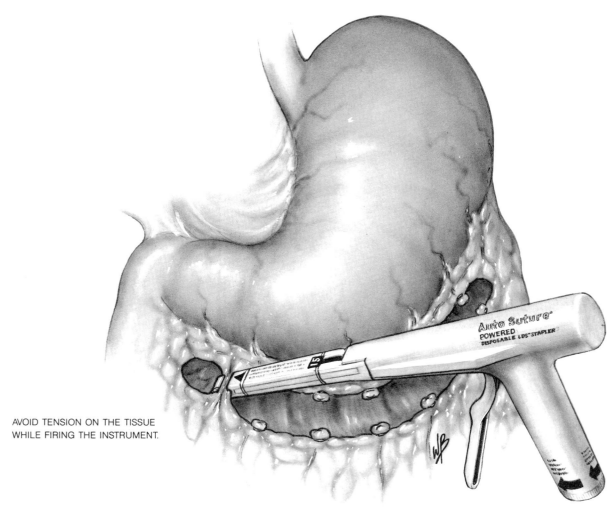

AVOID TENSION ON THE TISSUE
WHILE FIRING THE INSTRUMENT.

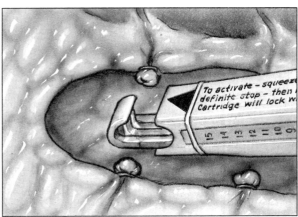

ASSURE THAT THE TISSUE AND STAPLES
ARE FREE OF THE CARTRIDGE PRIOR
TO REMOVING THE INSTRUMENT.

The stomach is mobilized using the LDS™ instrument to ligate and divide the omental vessels. Slip the tissue to be ligated into the jaw of the LDS™ instrument and fire the staples. Two staples ligate the vessel and a knife blade divides the vessel between the staples. To prevent incorporation of staples in the anastomosis, the LDS™ instrument may be used to within 2 cm. of the point of transection of the duodenum.

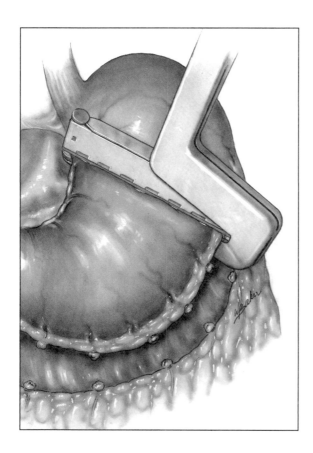

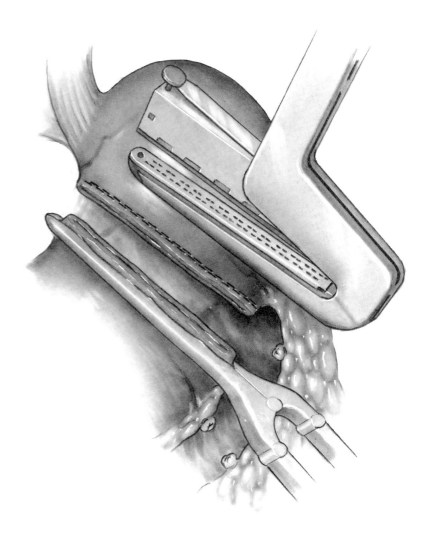

The TA® 90 instrument is used to close the gastric pouch. Slip the jaws of the instrument around the stomach at the level of transection, close the instrument and fire the staples. Before releasing the tissue, place a clamp on the specimen side and transect the stomach using the TA® 90 instrument edge as a cutting guide.

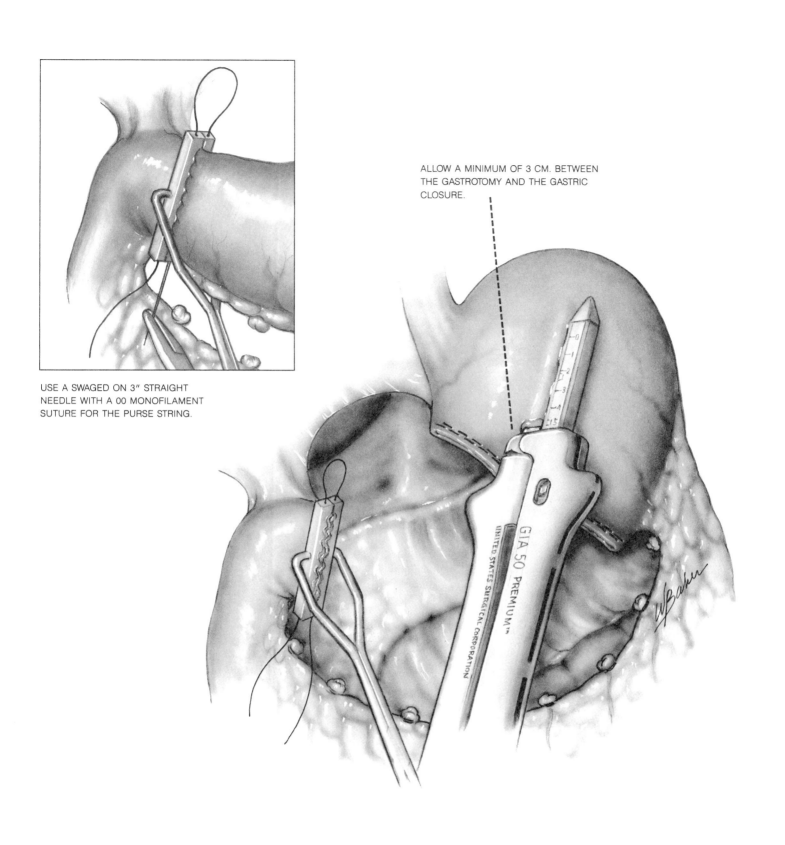

USE A SWAGED ON 3″ STRAIGHT
NEEDLE WITH A 00 MONOFILAMENT
SUTURE FOR THE PURSE STRING.

ALLOW A MINIMUM OF 3 CM. BETWEEN
THE GASTROTOMY AND THE GASTRIC
CLOSURE.

The purse string instrument is placed around the duodenum. Pass the suture through the superior jaw of the purse string instrument and return it through the inferior jaw. Place a clamp on the specimen side and use the purse string instrument edge as a cutting guide to transect the duodenum.

The purse string instrument is removed and the diameter of the duodenum is determined using the S-EEA™ sizers.

A gastrotomy is performed using the GIA™ instrument to incise the stomach and secure hemostasis of the cut edges. A 1 cm. stab wound is made into the anterior gastric wall. Insert the anvil fork of the instrument into the lumen of the stomach and place the cartridge fork on the serosal surface. Close the instrument and fire the staples. Two double staggered staple lines are placed in the anterior gastric wall and the knife in the instrument cuts an incision between them.

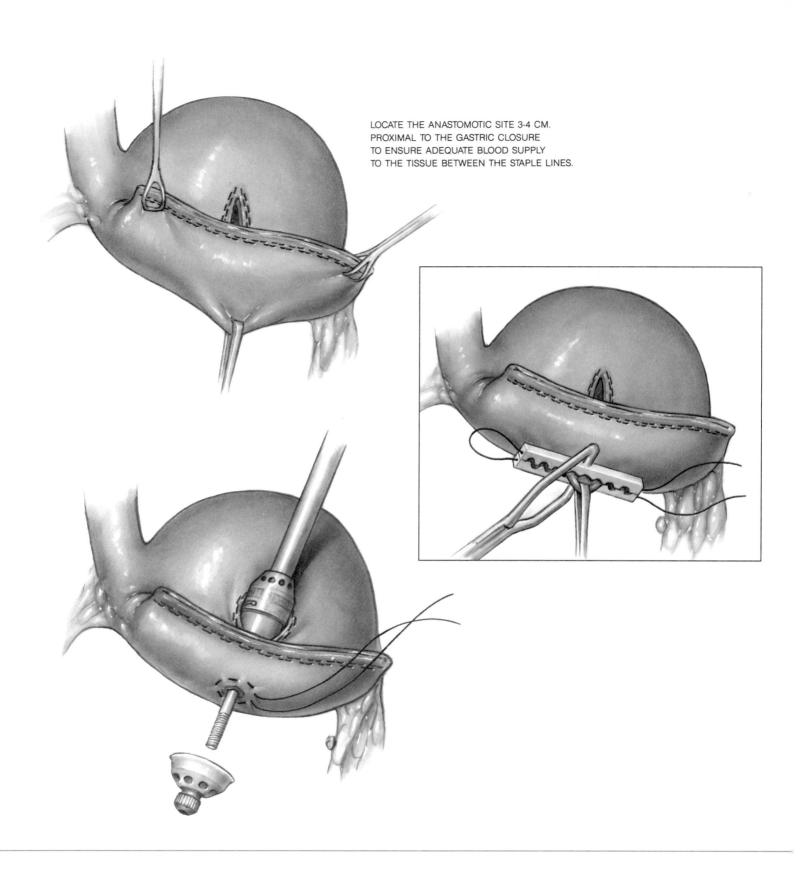

LOCATE THE ANASTOMOTIC SITE 3-4 CM.
PROXIMAL TO THE GASTRIC CLOSURE
TO ENSURE ADEQUATE BLOOD SUPPLY
TO THE TISSUE BETWEEN THE STAPLE LINES.

Identify the location of the anastomosis on the posterior gastric wall 3-4 cm. proximal to the gastric staple line closure. Grasp all tissue layers of the gastric wall with an Allis clamp. Apply the purse string instrument around the gastric tissue just beneath the Allis clamp and place a purse string suture. Excise the redundant tissue using the purse string instrument as a cutting guide.

The EEA™ instrument is used to create the anastomosis. Introduce the instrument, without anvil, into the lumen of the stomach. Place the tip of the center rod at the anastomotic site. Remove the purse string instrument, advance the center rod through the posterior gastric wall and tie the purse string suture. Place the anvil on the center rod.

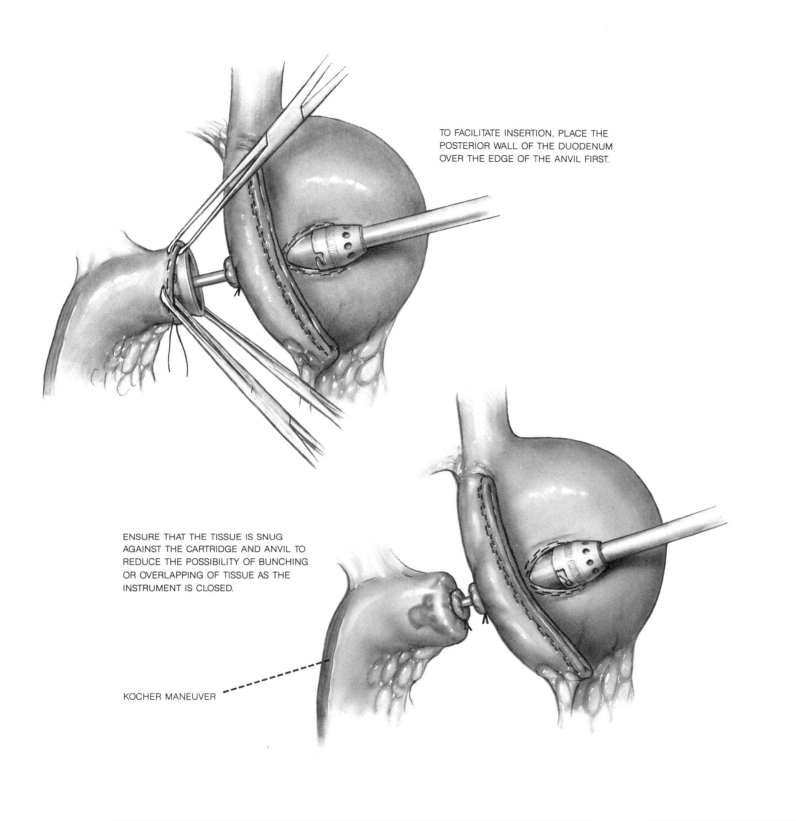

TO FACILITATE INSERTION, PLACE THE POSTERIOR WALL OF THE DUODENUM OVER THE EDGE OF THE ANVIL FIRST.

ENSURE THAT THE TISSUE IS SNUG AGAINST THE CARTRIDGE AND ANVIL TO REDUCE THE POSSIBILITY OF BUNCHING OR OVERLAPPING OF TISSUE AS THE INSTRUMENT IS CLOSED.

KOCHER MANEUVER

Grasp the duodenal edges with three Allis clamps placed equidistantly. Introduce the anvil into the duodenum, tie the purse string suture, close the EEA™ instrument and fire the staples. A circular double staggered row of staples joins the organs and the circular blade in the instrument cuts a stoma.

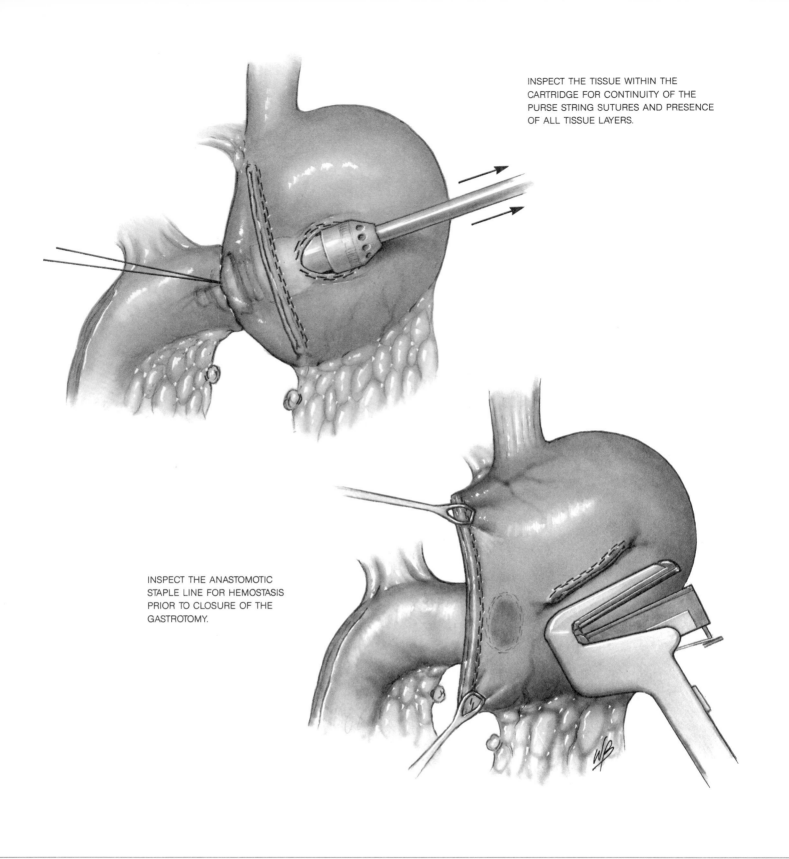

INSPECT THE TISSUE WITHIN THE
CARTRIDGE FOR CONTINUITY OF THE
PURSE STRING SUTURES AND PRESENCE
OF ALL TISSUE LAYERS.

INSPECT THE ANASTOMOTIC
STAPLE LINE FOR HEMOSTASIS
PRIOR TO CLOSURE OF THE
GASTROTOMY.

Open the instrument slightly and place a traction or figure-of-eight suture around the staple line. Lift the staple line over the anvil; simultaneously, gently rotate and remove the instrument.

Inspect the staple line for hemostasis prior to closing the gastrotomy with the TA® 55 instrument. Approxi-

mate the stapled tissue edges in an everted manner with Allis clamps or traction sutures. Slip the jaws of the TA® 55 instrument around the tissue, close the instrument and fire the staples. Before releasing the tissue, use the instrument edge as a guide to excise the margin of tissue protruding through the jaws.

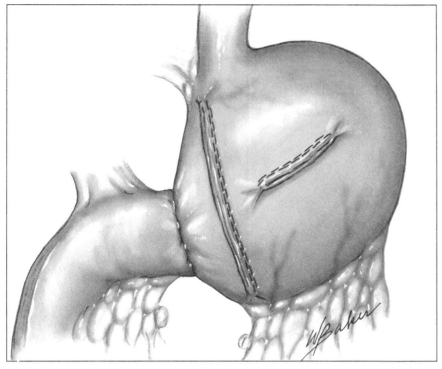

COMPLETED PROCEDURE

End-to-End Anastomosis

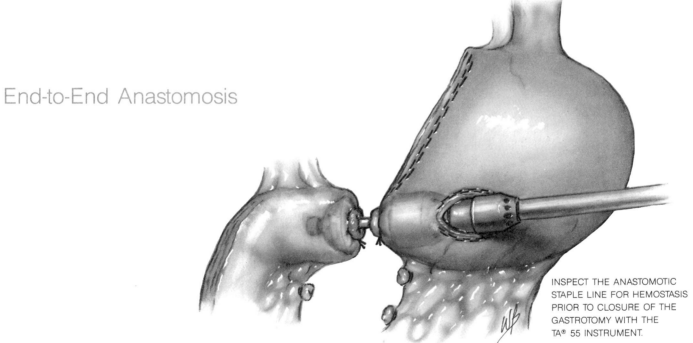

INSPECT THE ANASTOMOTIC STAPLE LINE FOR HEMOSTASIS PRIOR TO CLOSURE OF THE GASTROTOMY WITH THE TA® 55 INSTRUMENT.

An end-to-end gastroduodenostomy may be performed utilizing the greater curvature corner of the gastric closure. Introduce the EEA™ instrument, without anvil, through the gastrotomy. Excise the corner of the gastric staple line and place a manual purse string suture. Open the EEA™ instrument, advancing the center rod through the opening. Tie the purse string suture and place the anvil on the center rod. Introduce the anvil into the duodenum and tie the purse string suture. Complete the procedure as previously described.

Alternate Technique

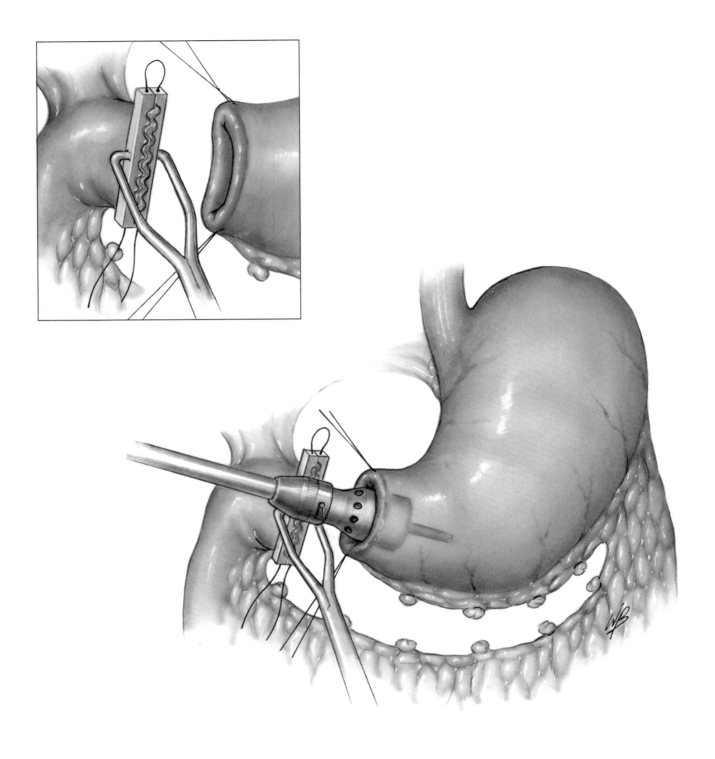

In gastric resection for benign pathology, the EEA™ instrument can be introduced into the stomach through the specimen.

The purse string suture is placed on the duodenum as previously described. Use the purse string

instrument edge as a cutting guide to transect the duodenum. Determine the diameter of the duodenum using the S-EEA™ sizers.

Introduce the EEA™ instrument, without anvil, through the open transected end of the stomach.

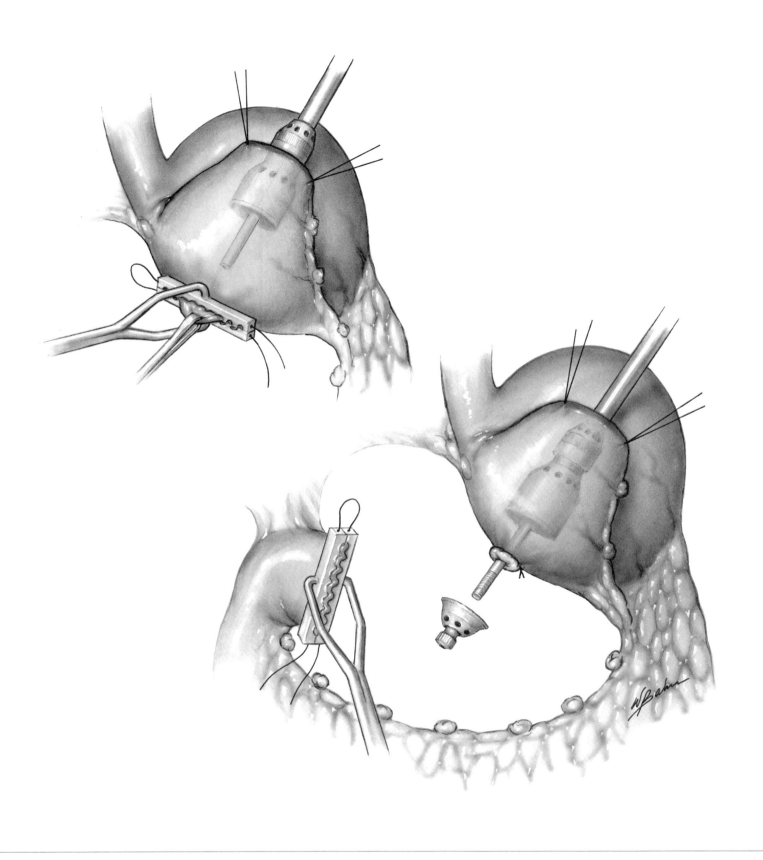

Identify the location of the anastomosis 3-4 cm. proximal to the proposed level of transection of the stomach. With an Allis clamp, grasp all tissue layers of the gastric wall. Apply the purse string instrument around the tissue just beneath the Allis clamp and place a purse string suture. Excise the redundant tissue using the purse string instrument as a cutting guide.

Remove the purse string instrument, advance the center rod through the gastric wall and tie the purse string suture. Place the anvil on the center rod.

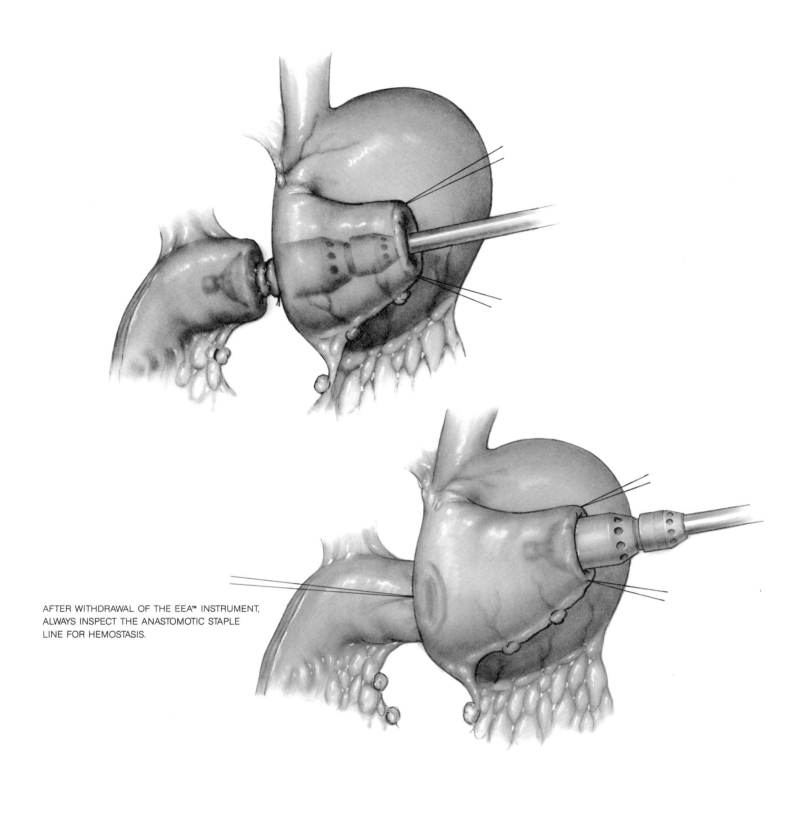

AFTER WITHDRAWAL OF THE EEA™ INSTRUMENT, ALWAYS INSPECT THE ANASTOMOTIC STAPLE LINE FOR HEMOSTASIS.

Introduce the anvil into the duodenum as previously described and tie the purse string suture. Close the EEA™ instrument and fire the staples.

Open the instrument slightly, gently rotate and remove the instrument. Always inspect the anastomotic staple line for hemostasis prior to closing the stomach.

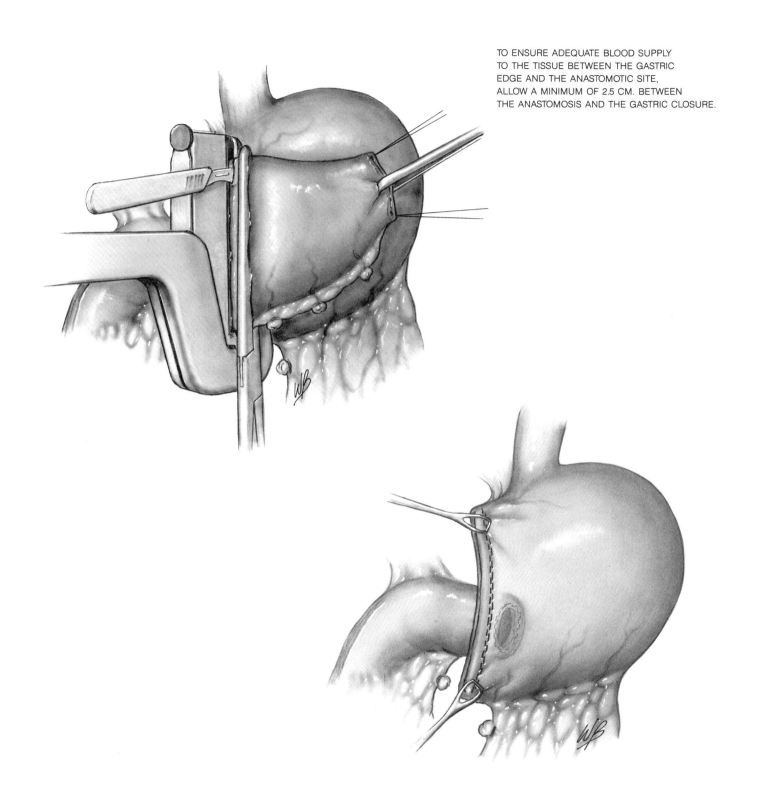

TO ENSURE ADEQUATE BLOOD SUPPLY
TO THE TISSUE BETWEEN THE GASTRIC
EDGE AND THE ANASTOMOTIC SITE,
ALLOW A MINIMUM OF 2.5 CM. BETWEEN
THE ANASTOMOSIS AND THE GASTRIC CLOSURE.

The TA® 90 instrument is used to close the gastric pouch. Slip the jaws of the instrument around the stomach at the level of transection, close the instrument and fire the staples. Resect the stomach using the instrument edge as a cutting guide.

The completed anastomosis is illustrated.

The fascia and skin are closed in the usual manner with the DFS™ instrument and the PREMIUM® skin stapler.

Total Gastrectomy and Esophagojejunostomy

Auto Suture® Instruments Used in a
Total Gastrectomy and Esophagojejunostomy with Roux-en-Y

See Cautions and Contraindications on page 236

INSTRUMENT	CLINICAL APPLICATION
LDS™ Instrument	Ligation and division of the omental vessels.
TA® 55 Instrument	Closure of the duodenum. Closure of the jejunotomy.
EEA™ Instrument or PREMIUM CEEA™ Instrument	Anastomosis of the jejunum to the esophagus. Anastomosis of the jejunum to the jejunum for the Roux-en-Y.
DFS™ Instrument and PREMIUM® Skin Stapler	Closure of fascia and skin.

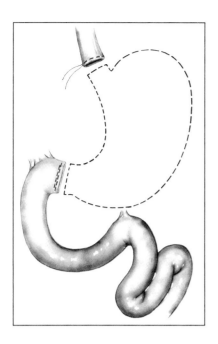

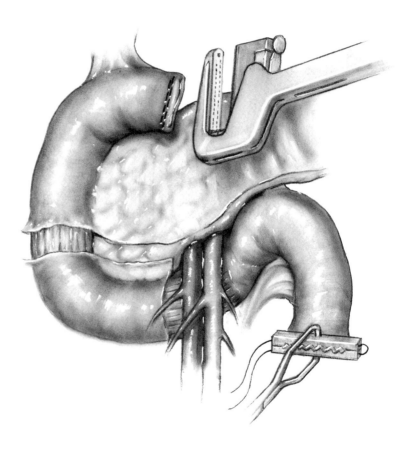

Total gastrectomy is performed using the LDS™ instrument to mobilize the stomach and the TA® 55 instrument to close the duodenum. Traction on the specimen facilitates placement of the purse string instrument and purse string suture on the esophagus prior to completing the gastric resection.

The jejunum is mobilized and transected 10-15 cm. distal to the ligament of Treitz. The purse string instrument is used to place a purse string suture on the proximal and distal cut edges.

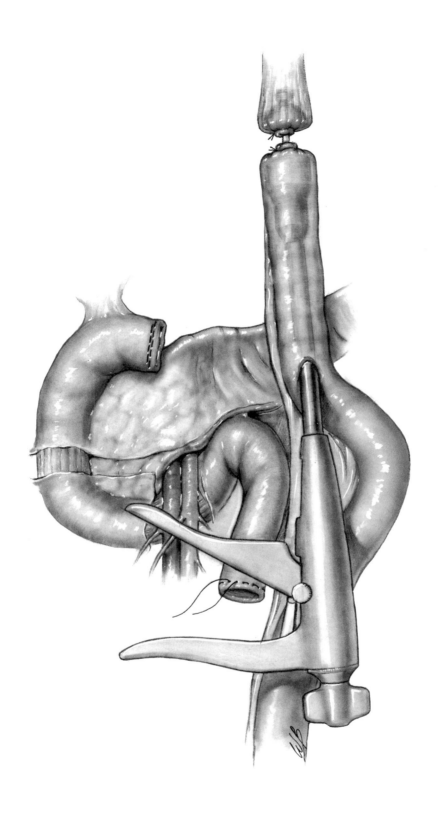

The EEA™ instrument is used to perform the esophagojejunostomy and the Roux-en-Y anastomosis. Introduce the instrument through an incision in the distal jejunum midway between the transected end and the selected site for the Roux-en-Y anastomosis. Advance the EEA™ instrument proximally to the level of the purse string suture. Open the instrument to advance the anvil and tie the purse string suture.

Introduce the anvil into the esophagus. The use of three Allis clamps or three traction sutures on the tissue edges facilitates insertion of the anvil. Tie the purse string suture, close the EEA™ instrument and fire the staples. Open the instrument slightly, gently rotate and remove the instrument.

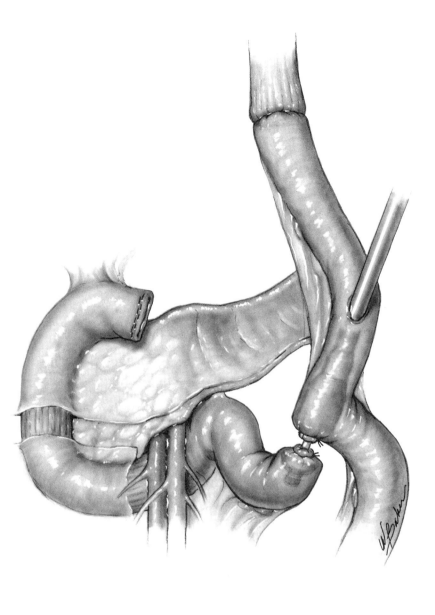

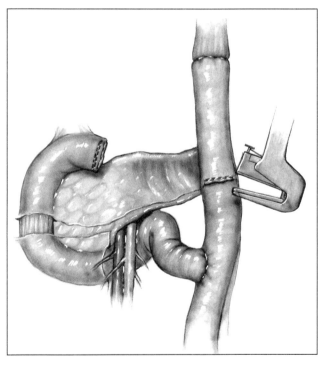

INSPECT THE ANASTOMOTIC STAPLE LINES FOR HEMOSTASIS
PRIOR TO TRANSVERSE CLOSURE OF THE JEJUNOTOMY.

Identify the site of the Roux-en-Y anastomosis on the distal jejunum. Introduce the EEA™ instrument, without anvil, through the jejunotomy and distally to the site of the anastomosis. Advance the center rod, tenting the tissue, and incise the jejunum over the center rod. Open the instrument to advance the center rod through the jejunal opening and place a manual purse string suture. Tie the suture and place the anvil on the center rod.

Introduce the anvil into the proximal jejunum and tie the purse string suture. Close the EEA™ instrument, fire the staples, and remove the instrument. Inspect the esophagojejunal and jejunojejunal anastomotic staple lines for hemostasis prior to transverse closure of the jejunotomy with the TA® 55 instrument.

The fascia and skin are closed in the usual manner with the DFS™ instrument and the PREMIUM® skin stapler.

Total Gastrectomy and Jejunal Interposition

Auto Suture® Instruments Used in a Total Gastrectomy and Jejunal Interposition

See Cautions and Contraindications on page 236

INSTRUMENT	CLINICAL APPLICATION
LDS™ Instrument	Ligation and division of the omental vessels.
GIA™ Instrument	Closure and transection of the proximal and distal jejunum. Anastomosis of the proximal and distal jejunum.
EEA™ Instrument or PREMIUM CEEA™ Instrument	Anastomosis of the jejunal segment to the esophagus. Anastomosis of the jejunal segment to the duodenum.
TA® 55 Instrument	Closure of the jejunotomy. Closure of the common stab wounds.
DFS™ Instrument and PREMIUM® Skin Stapler	Closure of fascia and skin.

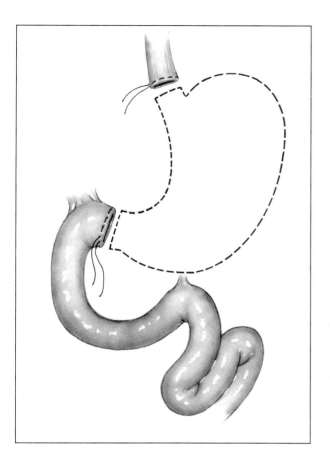

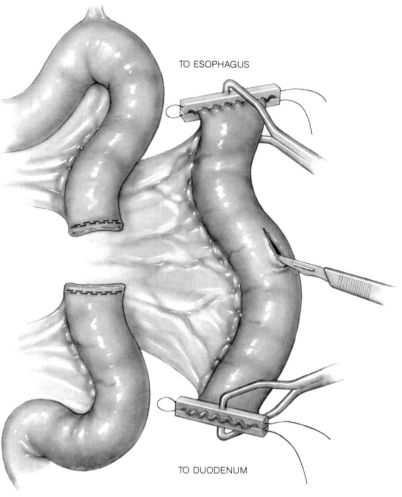

TO ESOPHAGUS

TO DUODENUM

Total gastrectomy is performed using the LDS™ instrument to mobilize the stomach. The esophagus and duodenum are prepared with purse string sutures and the stomach is resected.

The jejunal segment for interposition is identified and the proximal and distal jejunum are closed and transected using the GIA™ instrument. The jejunal segment is prepared with purse string sutures. Place the purse string instrument around the proximal end of the jejunal segment just beneath the staple line closure.

Apply the purse string suture and excise the redundant tissue using the purse string instrument as a cutting guide. Repeat the procedure on the distal end of the jejunal segment.

Following determination of the diameter of the esophagus and the duodenum using the S-EEA™ sizers, a 2.5-3 cm. incision is made in the anti-mesenteric border of the jejunal segment midway between the purse string sutures.

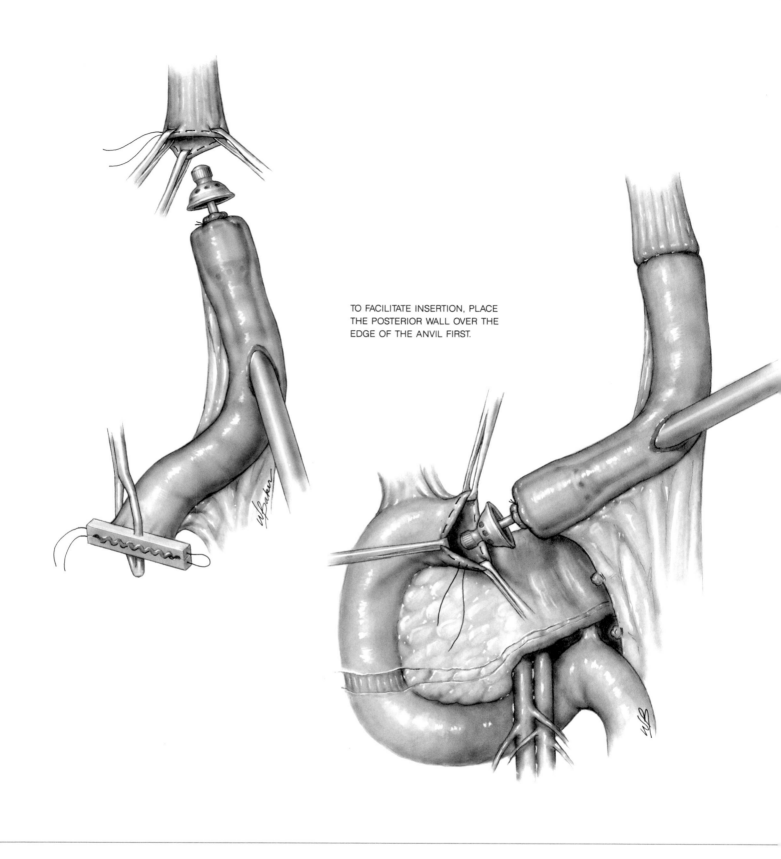

TO FACILITATE INSERTION, PLACE
THE POSTERIOR WALL OVER THE
EDGE OF THE ANVIL FIRST.

The EEA™ instrument is used to perform the esophagojejunostomy and the jejunoduodenostomy. Introduce the EEA™ instrument into the jejunum and advance it proximally to the level of the purse string instrument. Remove the purse string instrument and open the EEA™ instrument advancing the anvil. Tie the purse string suture.

Grasp the tissue edges of the esophagus with three Allis clamps placed equidistantly. Introduce the anvil into the esophagus and tie the purse string suture. Close the instrument and fire the staples. Open the instrument slightly; simultaneously, gently rotate and remove the instrument. Repeat the procedure for the jejunoduodenostomy.

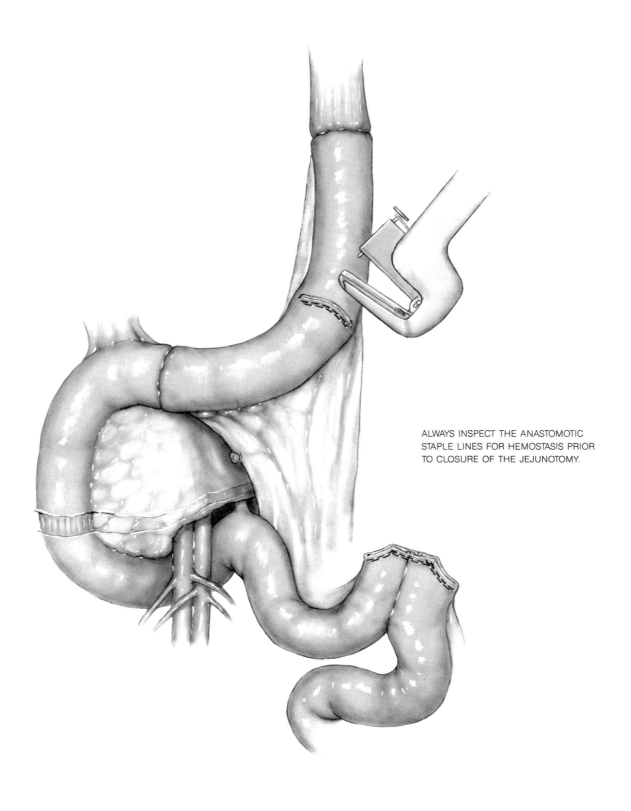

ALWAYS INSPECT THE ANASTOMOTIC
STAPLE LINES FOR HEMOSTASIS PRIOR
TO CLOSURE OF THE JEJUNOTOMY.

Inspect the anastomoses for hemostasis prior to transverse closure of the jejunotomy with the TA® 55 instrument.

Intestinal continuity is re-established by performing a functional end-to-end anastomosis.

The fascia and skin are closed in the usual manner with the DFS™ instrument and the PREMIUM® skin stapler.

Paulino Gastric Substitute

Auto Suture® Instruments Used in a Total Gastrectomy and Paulino Gastric Substitute

See Cautions and Contraindications on page 236

INSTRUMENT	CLINICAL APPLICATION
LDS™ Instrument	Ligation and division of the omental vessels.
TA® 55 Instrument	Closure of the duodenum. Closure of the common stab wounds. Closure of the jejunum.
GIA™ Instrument	Closure and transection of the jejunum. Anastomosis of the jejunal segments forming the pouch.
EEA™ Instrument or PREMIUM CEEA™ Instrument	Anastomosis of the esophagus to the isoperistaltic jejunal segment.
DFS™ Instrument and PREMIUM® Skin Stapler	Closure of fascia and skin.

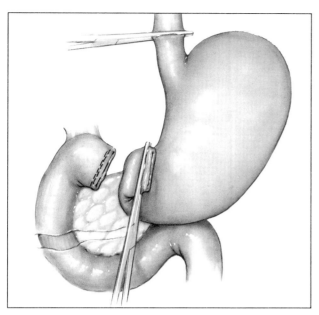

PERFORM THE ESOPHAGEAL TRANSECTION AGAINST
A KOCHER CLAMP DISTAL TO DESIRED
ANASTOMOTIC SITE.

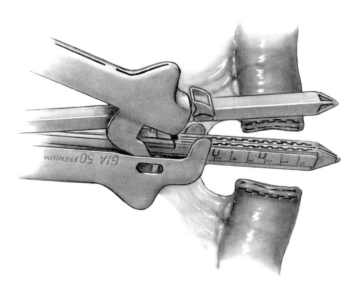

PERFORM THE JEJUNAL TRANSECTION
20-25 CM. DISTAL TO LIG. OF TREITZ.

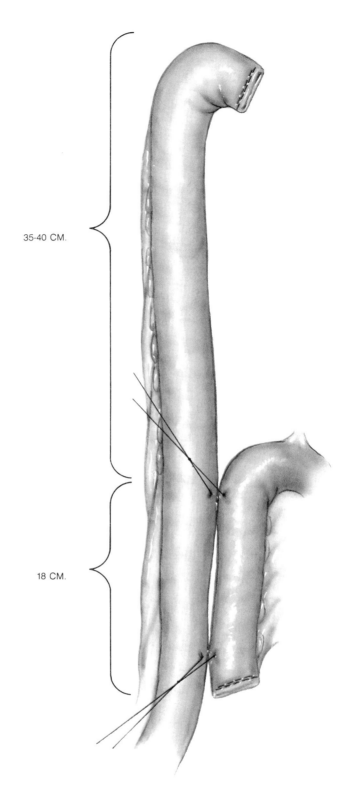

35-40 CM.

18 CM.

Total gastrectomy is performed using the LDS™
instrument to ligate and divide the omental vessels
and the TA® 55 instrument to close the duodenum.

The jejunum is closed and transected using the GIA™
instrument. Place the instrument around the jejunum
20-25 cm. distal to the ligament of Treitz. Close the
instrument and fire the staples. Two double staggered
staple lines seal the jejunum; simultaneously, a knife

blade in the instrument transects the jejunum between
the two double staple lines.

The jejunal segment leading from the esophagus to
the Paulino gastric substitute should measure 35-40
cm. and the pouch 18 cm. With the aid of traction
sutures, approximate the antimesenteric borders of the
jejunum in a Roux-en-Y fashion.

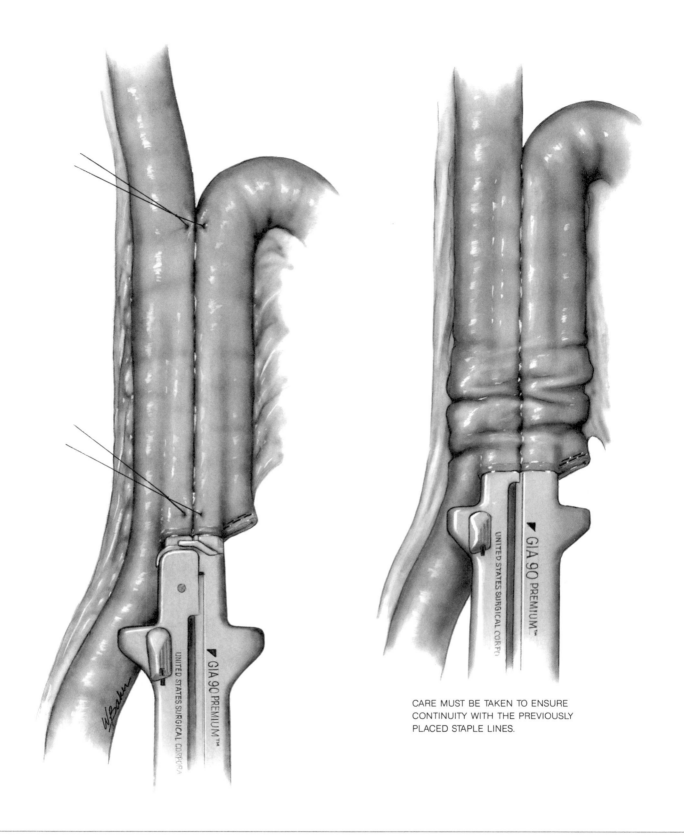

CARE MUST BE TAKEN TO ENSURE
CONTINUITY WITH THE PREVIOUSLY
PLACED STAPLE LINES.

The Paulino gastric substitute is created with the GIA™ instrument. Excise the antimesenteric corner of the proximal jejunal segment and make a stab wound in the antimesenteric border of the apposed jejunum. Insert one fork of the instrument into each lumen, close the instrument and fire the staples.

The pouch is completed with repeated application of the instrument through the same common opening. Care must be taken to incorporate the end staples of the previous application to ensure continuity of the staple lines.

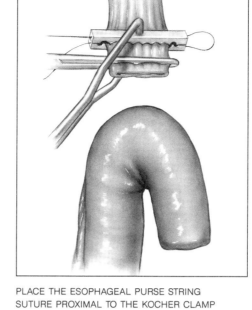

PLACE THE ESOPHAGEAL PURSE STRING
SUTURE PROXIMAL TO THE KOCHER CLAMP
AND EXCISE THE EXCESS TISSUE.

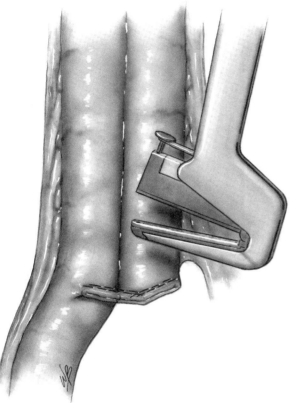

CARE MUST BE TAKEN TO
OVERLAP THE ENDS OF THE
PREVIOUS STAPLE LINES.

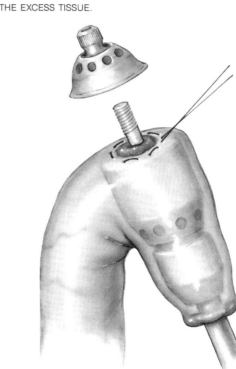

Always inspect the anastomotic staple lines for
hemostasis prior to closing the common opening with
the TA® 55 instrument.

The EEA™ instrument is used to perform the
esophagojejunal anastomosis. Place a purse string
suture on the esophagus and excise the excess tissue
using the purse string instrument as a cutting guide.

Excise the staple line on the jejunum and identify the
site of the anastomosis. Introduce the EEA™
instrument, without anvil, into the jejunum. Advance
the center rod through an antimesenteric stab wound
surrounded by a purse string suture. Tie the suture
and place the anvil on the center rod.

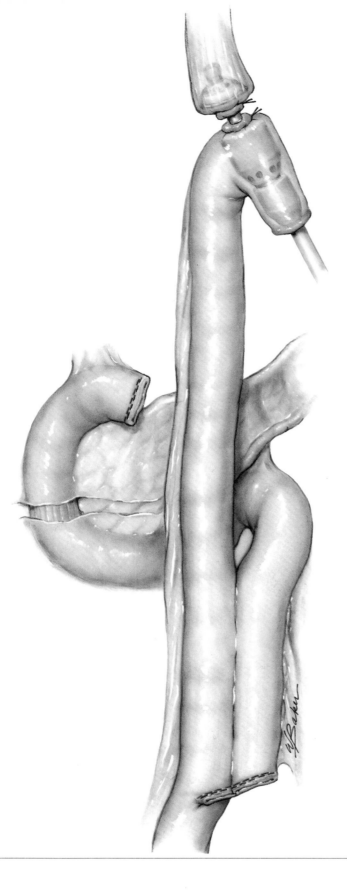

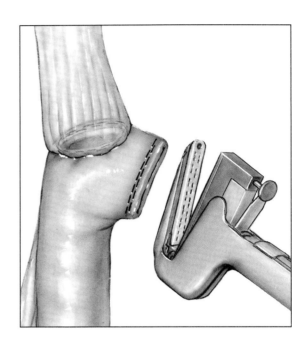

ENSURE THAT THE TISSUE IS SNUG
AGAINST THE CARTRIDGE AND ANVIL TO
REDUCE THE POSSIBILITY OF BUNCHING
OR OVERLAPPING OF TISSUE AS THE
INSTRUMENT IS CLOSED.

Remove the purse string instrument and grasp the esophageal edges with three Allis clamps or sutures placed equidistantly. Introduce the anvil into the esophagus, tie the purse string suture, close the EEA™ instrument and fire the staples. Open the instrument slightly and place a traction or figure-of-eight suture around the staple line. Lift the staple line over the anvil; simultaneously, gently rotate and remove the instrument. Check the anastomosis for hemostasis before closing the jejunum with the TA® 55 instrument.

Alternate Technique

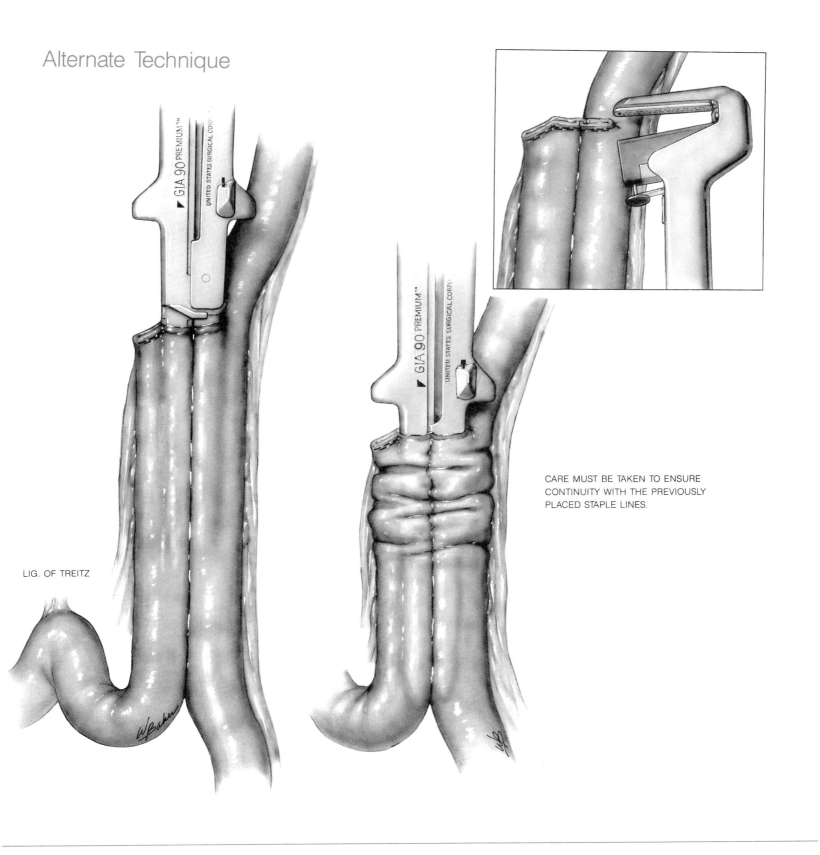

LIG. OF TREITZ

CARE MUST BE TAKEN TO ENSURE
CONTINUITY WITH THE PREVIOUSLY
PLACED STAPLE LINES.

The pouch may be created by approximating the proximal jejunal segment in an antiperistaltic fashion along the right side of the distal jejunal segment. The pouch is created by serial applications of the GIA™ instrument. Take care to incorporate the end staples of the previous application to ensure continuity of the staple lines.

Inspect the anastomotic staple lines for hemostasis prior to closing the common opening with the TA® 55 instrument.

The fascia and skin are closed in the usual manner with the DFS™ instrument and the PREMIUM® skin stapler.

Auto Suture® Instruments Used in a
Total Gastrectomy and Hunt Lawrence Pouch

See Cautions and Contraindications on page 236

INSTRUMENT	CLINICAL APPLICATION
LDS™ Instrument	Ligation and division of the omental vessels.
TA® 55 Instrument	Closure of the duodenum. Closure of the common stab wounds.
GIA™ Instrument	Closure and transection of the jejunum. Anastomosis of the jejunal loop forming the pouch. Anastomosis of the proximal and distal jejunum for the Roux-en-Y.
PREMIUM CEEA™ Instrument or EEA™ Instrument	Anastomosis of the jejunal pouch to the esophagus.
DFS™ Instrument and PREMIUM® Skin Stapler	Closure of fascia and skin.

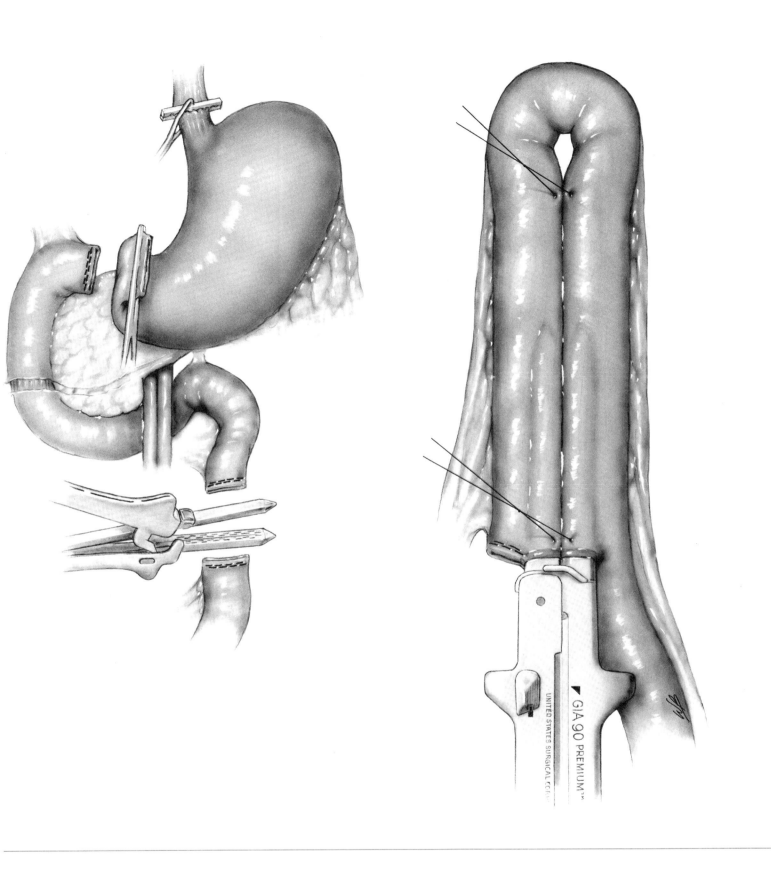

Total gastrectomy is performed using the LDS™ instrument to mobilize the stomach. The duodenum is closed with the TA® 55 instrument and the esophagus is prepared with a purse string suture prior to transection. The jejunum is closed and transected using the GIA™ instrument.

The distal jejunum is looped on itself for a distance of 15-20 cm. and the antimesenteric borders are approximated with traction sutures. The GIA™ instrument is used to create the pouch. Excise the antimesenteric corner of the staple line closure and make a

corresponding stab wound in the antimesenteric border of the apposed jejunum. Insert one fork of the GIA™ instrument into each lumen. Close the instrument and fire the staples.

The pouch is completed with repeated application of the instrument through the same common opening. A jejunojejunal spur is left in the apical portion of the pouch. Care must be taken to incorporate the end staples of the previous application to ensure continuity of the staple lines. Inspect the anastomotic staple lines for hemostasis.

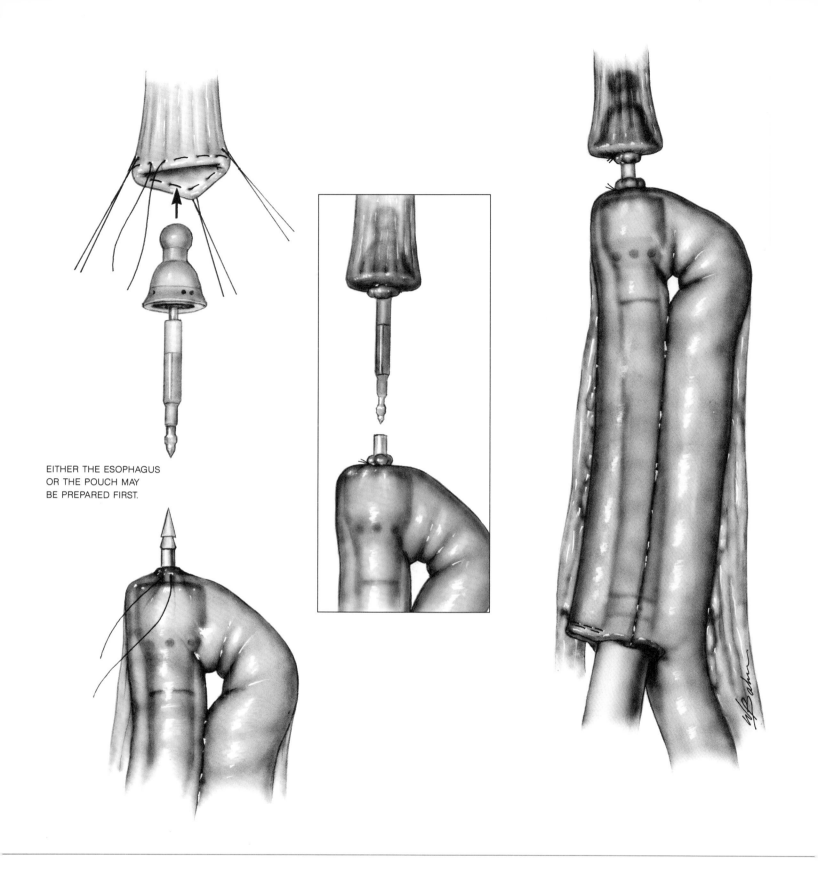

EITHER THE ESOPHAGUS
OR THE POUCH MAY
BE PREPARED FIRST.

The esophagojejunostomy is performed using the PREMIUM CEEA™ instrument. Introduce the instrument, without anvil and anvil shaft and with recessed trocar tip, into the pouch and advance the instrument proximally to the site of anastomosis. Advance the trocar tip to perforate the jejunum and place a manual purse string suture around the instrument shaft. Tie the suture and remove the trocar tip with a Babcock clamp.

Remove the purse string instrument on the esophagus and grasp the esophageal edges with three traction sutures or Allis clamps placed equidistantly. Introduce the anvil with anvil shaft into the esophagus and tie the purse string suture. Engage the anvil shaft in the instrument shaft. Close the instrument and fire the staples. Open the instrument slightly; simultaneously, gently rotate and remove the instrument. Inspect the anastomosis for hemostasis prior to closure of the common stab wound with the TA® 55 instrument.

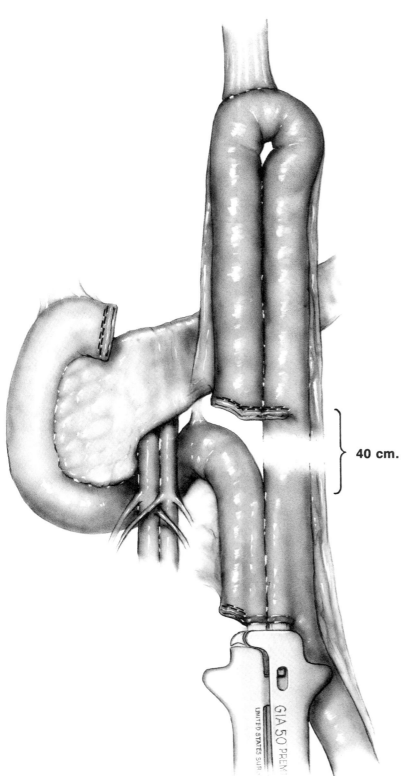

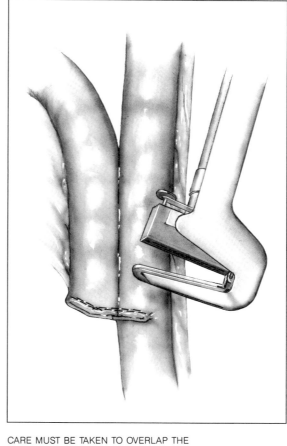

40 cm.

CARE MUST BE TAKEN TO OVERLAP THE
ENDS OF THE PREVIOUS STAPLE LINES.

The proximal jejunum is approximated to the efferent jejunum in a Roux-en-Y fashion 35-40 cm. distal to the pouch. The GIA™ instrument is used to perform the jejunojejunostomy. Excise the antimesenteric corner of the staple line closure and make a corresponding stab wound in the antimesenteric border of the apposed jejunum. Insert one fork of the instrument into each lumen, close the instrument and fire the staples.

Inspect the anastomotic staple lines for hemostasis prior to closure of the common stab wound with the TA® 55 instrument.

The fascia and skin are closed in the usual manner with the DFS™ instrument and the PREMIUM® skin stapler.

Gastrostomy

Auto Suture® Instruments
Used in a Gastrostomy

See Cautions and Contraindications on page 236

INSTRUMENT	CLINICAL APPLICATION
LDS™ Instrument	Ligation and division of the omental vessels in a continent gastrostomy.
GIA™ Instrument	Creation of the gastrostomy tube.
DFS™ Instrument and PREMIUM® Skin Stapler	Closure of fascia and skin.

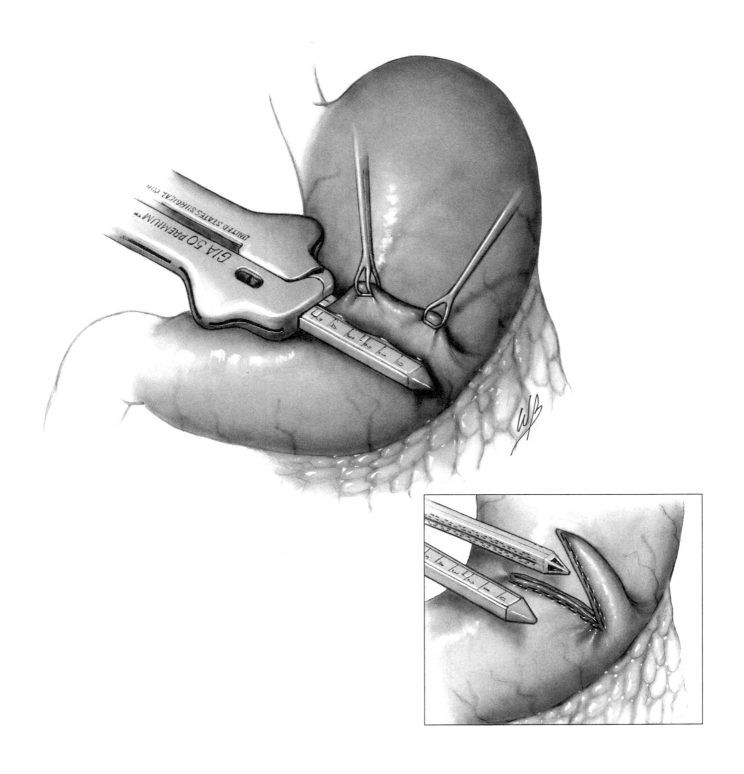

A tube of the anterior gastric wall is created with the GIA™ instrument. The anterior gastric wall is grasped with two Babcock clamps and drawn upward. Apply the GIA™ instrument to the serosal surface of the stomach with the tip of the forks 3 cm. from the greater curvature. Close the instrument and fire the staples. A double staggered staple line seals the anterior gastric wall and a second double staggered staple line seals the newly created gastric tube. Simultaneously, the knife blade in the instrument divides between the two double staple lines separating the gastric tube from the stomach. The proximal end of the gastric tube remains closed, which minimizes intraperitoneal contamination.

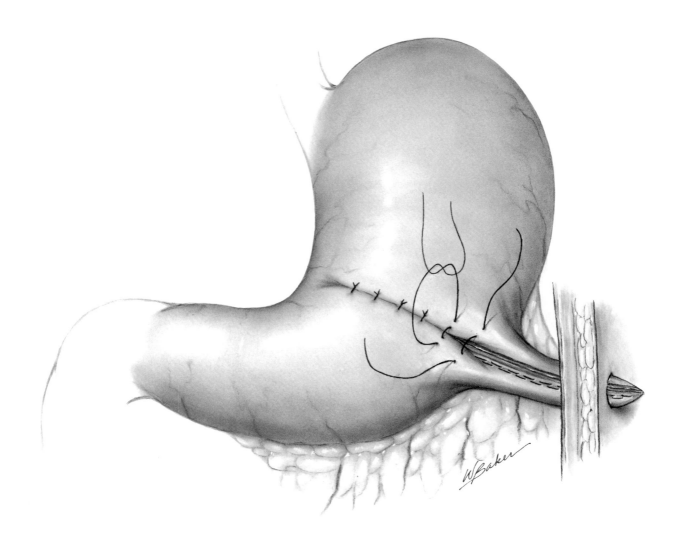

The staple line in this procedure is inverted with interrupted silk sutures taking care not to decrease the diameter of the tube.

The gastric tube is brought out through a stab wound in the abdominal wall. Seromuscular sutures are placed to secure the gastric tube and the tip of the gastric tube is amputated.

Continent Gastrostomy

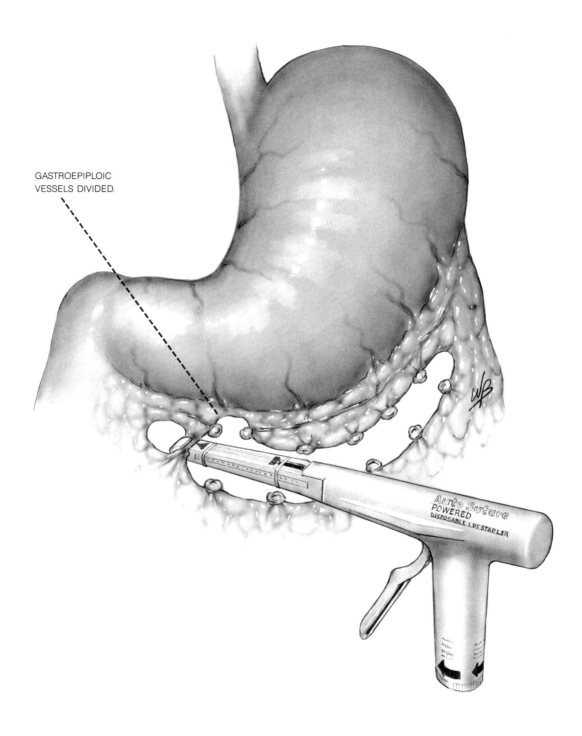

GASTROEPIPLOIC
VESSELS DIVIDED.

The greater curvature of the stomach is mobilized using the LDS™ instrument to ligate and divide the gastrocolic omentum peripheral to the gastroepiploic vessels. The right gastroepiploic artery is divided at the beginning point of the gastric tube to be constructed.

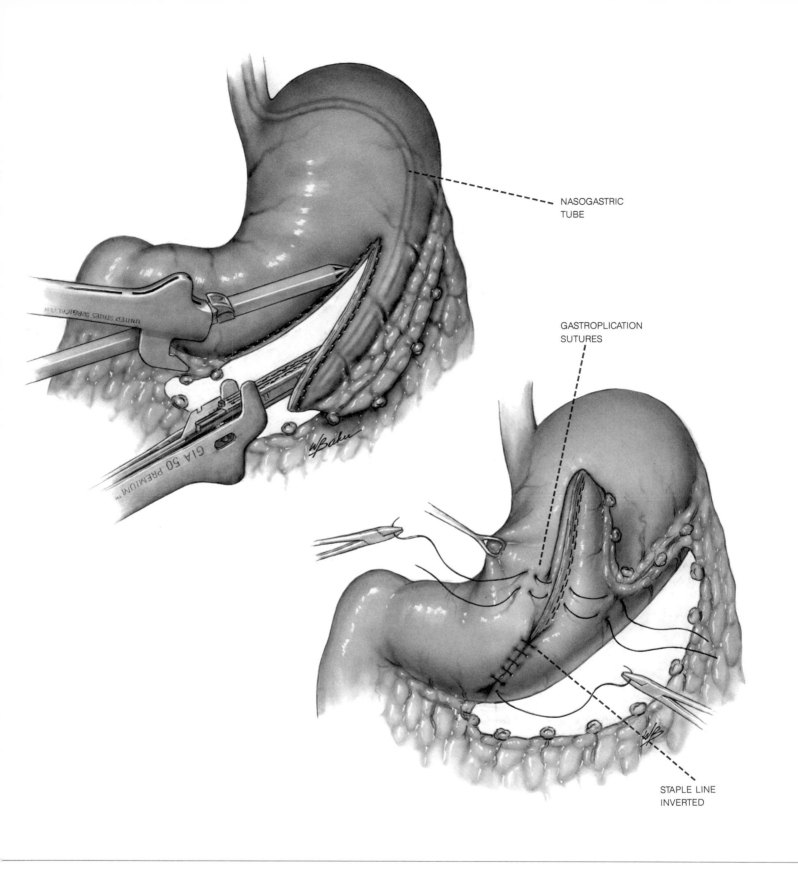

NASOGASTRIC
TUBE

GASTROPLICATION
SUTURES

STAPLE LINE
INVERTED

A bougie or nasogastric tube is passed and placed along the greater curvature of the stomach as a transection guide. The gastric tube is created by two applications of the GIA™ instrument. In this procedure, it is recommended that the staple line be oversewn and inverted with a continuous whip stitch or interrupted sutures.

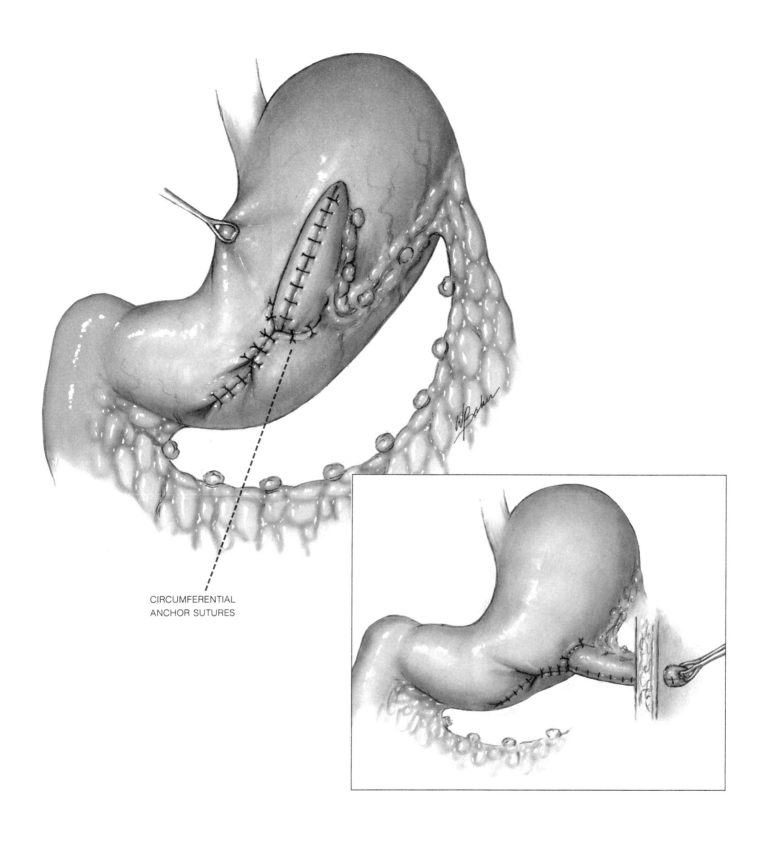

CIRCUMFERENTIAL
ANCHOR SUTURES

Gastroplication and circumferential anchor sutures are placed to support the gastrostomy and provide an antireflux mechanism.

The gastric tube is brought out through the abdominal wall and seromuscular sutures are placed to secure the tube. The tip of the gastric tube is excised and the mucosa sutured flush to the skin, completing the gastrostomy.

The fascia and skin are closed in the usual manner with the DFS™ instrument and the PREMIUM® skin stapler.

Excision of Gastric Wall Lesion

Auto Suture® Instruments Used for Excision of a Gastric Wall Lesion

See Cautions and Contraindications on page 236

INSTRUMENT	CLINICAL APPLICATION
LDS™ Instrument	Ligation and division of the omental vessels.
TA® 90 Instrument	Excision of the gastric wall lesion.
DFS™ Instrument and PREMIUM® Skin Stapler	Closure of fascia and skin.

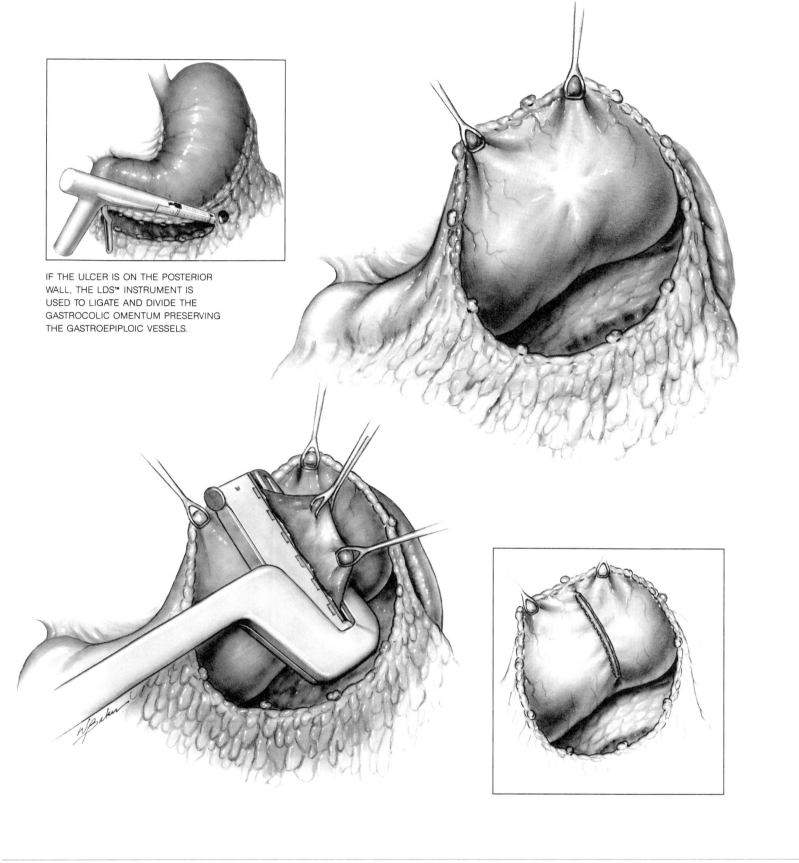

IF THE ULCER IS ON THE POSTERIOR WALL, THE LDS™ INSTRUMENT IS USED TO LIGATE AND DIVIDE THE GASTROCOLIC OMENTUM PRESERVING THE GASTROEPIPLOIC VESSELS.

The greater curvature is elevated to expose the posterior gastric wall. The gastric wall surrounding the lesion is grasped with two Babcock clamps and drawn upward. Incorporate the tissue within the jaws of the TA® 90 instrument. Close the instrument and fire the staples. Use the TA® 90 instrument edge as a cutting guide to excise the lesion.

The fascia and skin are closed in the usual manner with the DFS™ instrument and the PREMIUM® skin stapler.

Posterior Retrocolic Gastroenterostomy

Auto Suture® Instruments Used in a Posterior Retrocolic Gastroenterostomy

See Cautions and Contraindications on page 236

INSTRUMENT	CLINICAL APPLICATION
GIA™ Instrument	Anastomosis of the jejunum to the stomach.
TA® 55 Instrument	Closure of the gastrojejunal stab wound.
DFS™ Instrument and PREMIUM® Skin Stapler	Closure of fascia and skin.

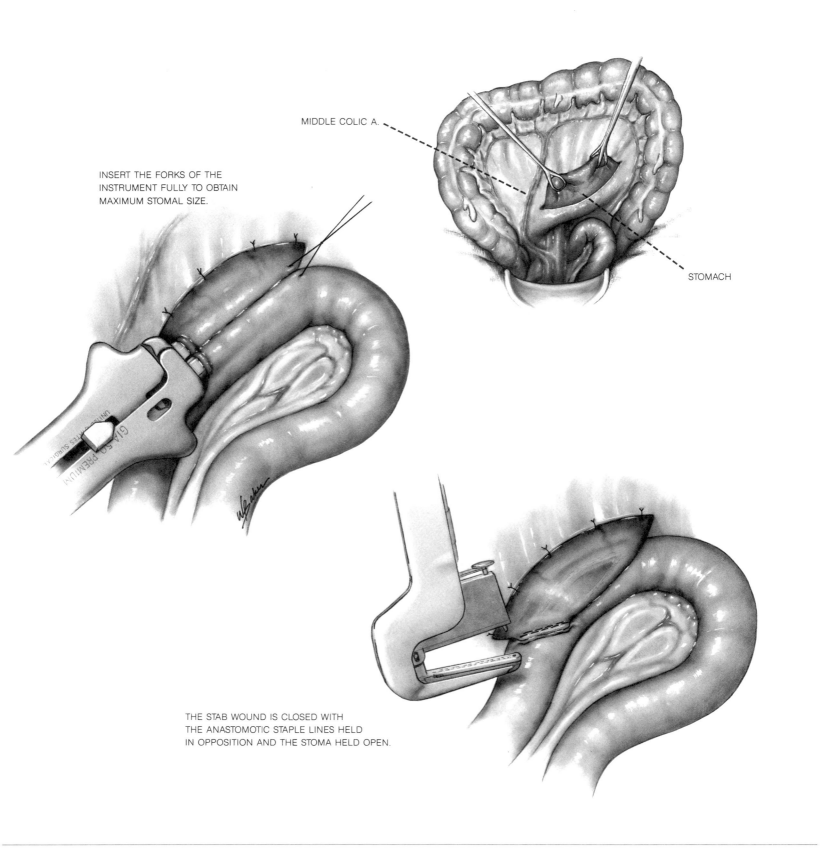

INSERT THE FORKS OF THE
INSTRUMENT FULLY TO OBTAIN
MAXIMUM STOMAL SIZE.

MIDDLE COLIC A.

STOMACH

THE STAB WOUND IS CLOSED WITH
THE ANASTOMOTIC STAPLE LINES HELD
IN OPPOSITION AND THE STOMA HELD OPEN.

The posterior wall of the stomach, proximal and close to the pylorus, is drawn through an avascular rent in the transverse mesocolon and sutured to the mesenteric margins.

The antimesenteric border of an appropriately selected proximal loop of jejunum is approximated to the gastric wall with traction sutures.

The bypass gastroenterostomy is performed using the GIA™ instrument. Make a 1 cm. stab wound into the

lumen of the stomach and a corresponding stab wound into the lumen of the jejunum. Insert one fork of the GIA™ instrument into each lumen, close the instrument and fire the staples.

Inspect the anastomotic staple lines for hemostasis prior to closure of the now common stab wound with the TA® 55 instrument.

The fascia and skin are closed in the usual manner with the DFS™ instrument and the PREMIUM® skin stapler.

Gastric Bypass

Auto Suture® Instruments Used in a Gastric Bypass with Roux-en-Y

See Cautions and Contraindications on page 236

INSTRUMENT	CLINICAL APPLICATION
TA 90 B™ Instrument	Closure of the gastric pouch.
GIA™ Instrument	Closure and transection of the jejunum. Anastomosis of the distal jejunum to the gastric fundus. Anastomosis of the proximal and distal jejunum.
TA® 55 Instrument	Closure of the jejunal stab wounds.
DFS™ Instrument and PREMIUM® Skin Stapler	Closure of fascia and skin.

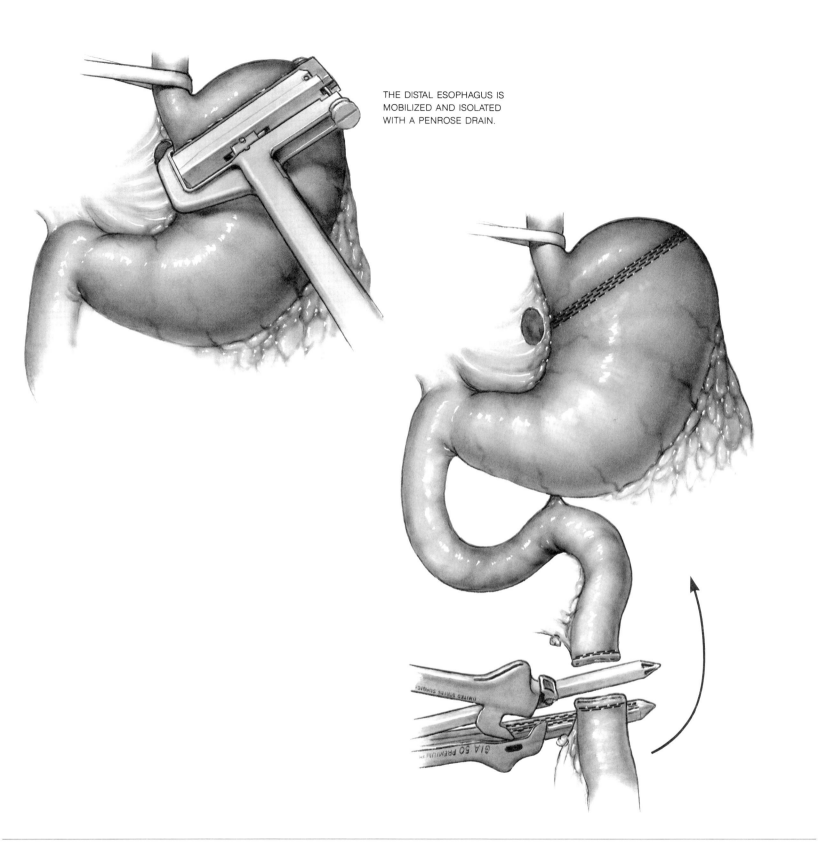

THE DISTAL ESOPHAGUS IS
MOBILIZED AND ISOLATED
WITH A PENROSE DRAIN.

The gastric partition is created with the TA 90 B™
instrument. Make an opening in the lesser omentum
at the level of the partition. Apply the TA 90 B™
instrument across the stomach from the lesser to the
greater curvature. Close the instrument, measure the
pouch volume and fire the staples. Four staggered
rows of staples partition the stomach.

The GIA™ instrument is used to close and transect the
jejunum. Place the instrument around the jejunum at
the point of transection in a scissor-like fashion, close
the instrument and fire the staples. Two double
staggered rows of staples seal the jejunum;
simultaneously, the knife blade in the instrument
transects the jejunum between the two double staple
lines.

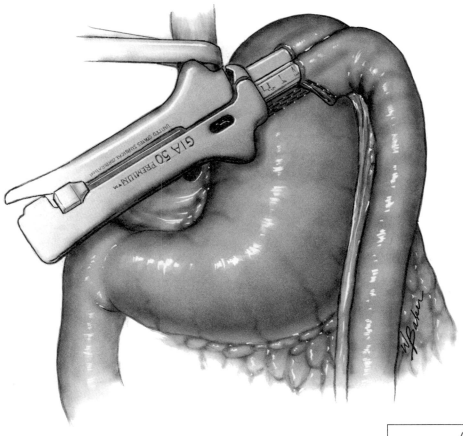

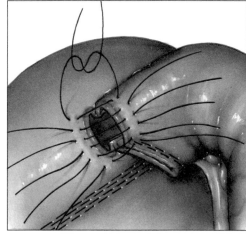

INSPECT THE ANASTOMOSIS FOR HEMOSTASIS PRIOR
TO MANUAL CLOSURE OF THE COMMON STAB WOUND.

The gastrojejunostomy is performed with the GIA™ instrument. Approximate the antimesenteric border of the distal jejunum to the fundus of the stomach 2.5 cm. from the gastric staple lines and 2.5 cm. from the greater curvature. Make a 1 cm. stab wound into the lumen of the gastric fundus and excise the anti-mesenteric corner of the staple line closure of the jejunum. Insert the cartridge fork of the instrument into the lumen of the jejunum and the anvil fork into the lumen of the stomach. Insert the forks of the GIA™ instrument approximately 2-3 cm. Close the instrument and fire the staples. Inspect the anastomosis for hemostasis prior to manual closure of the now common stab wound.

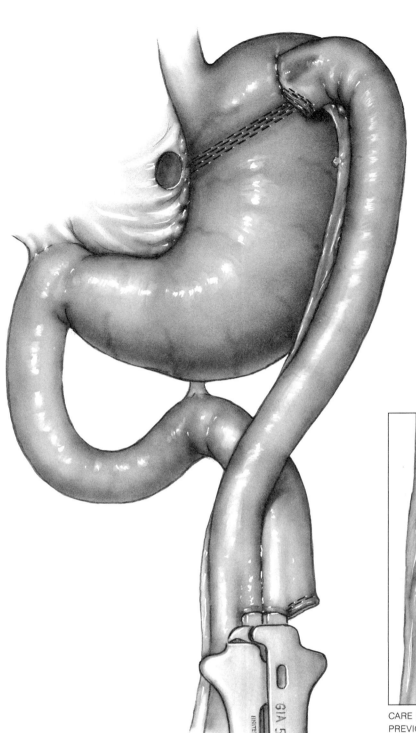

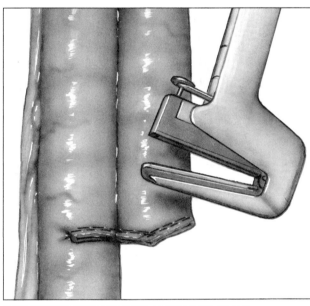

CARE MUST BE TAKEN TO OVERLAP THE ENDS OF THE PREVIOUS STAPLE LINES.

The GIA™ instrument is used to perform the Roux-en-Y anastomosis. Excise the antimesenteric corner of the proximal jejunum and make a 1 cm. stab wound into the antimesenteric border of the apposed jejunum. Insert one fork of the instrument into each lumen. Close the instrument and fire the staples. Inspect the anastomotic staple lines for hemostasis prior to closing the common opening with the TA® 55 instrument.

The fascia and skin are closed in the usual manner with the DFS™ instrument and the PREMIUM® skin stapler.

Vertical Banded Gastroplasty

Auto Suture® Instruments Used in a
Vertical Banded Gastroplasty

See Cautions and Contraindications on page 236

INSTRUMENT	CLINICAL APPLICATION
PREMIUM CEEA™ Instrument	Creation of the gastric window.
TA 90 B™ Instrument	Partition of the gastric pouch
DFS™ Instrument and PREMIUM® Skin Stapler	Closure of fascia and skin.

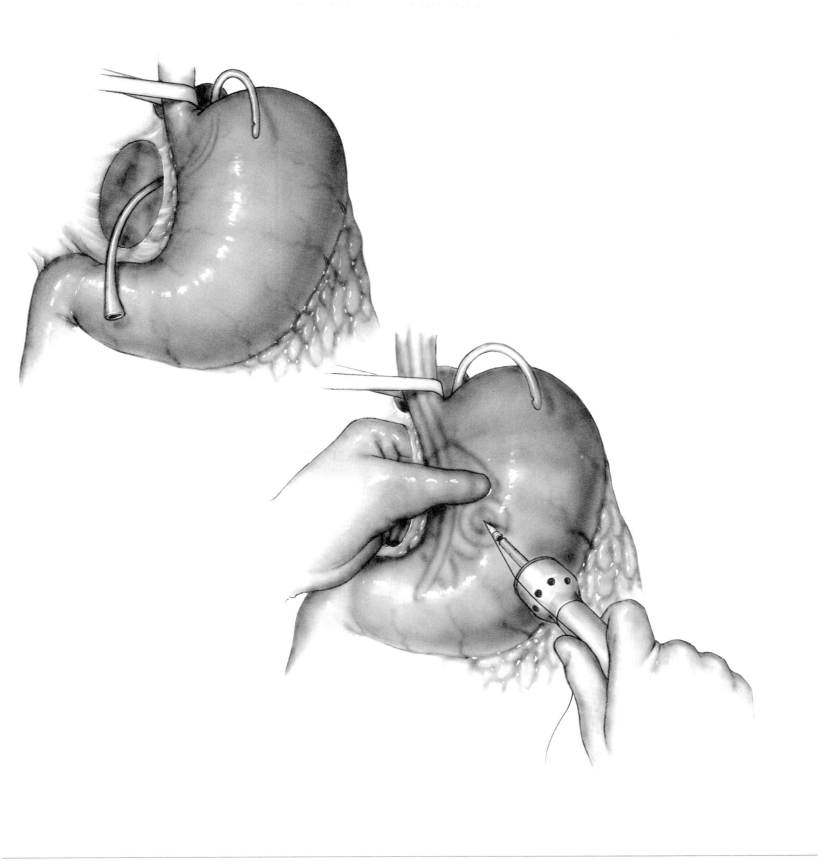

The distal esophagus is mobilized and isolated with a Penrose drain. An opening is made in the lesser omentum and a catheter is passed from the opening to the angle of His.

The PREMIUM CEEA™ instrument is used to create a gastric window 8-9 cm. distal to the esophagogastric junction and parallel to the lesser curvature of the stomach. Place the anvil of the PREMIUM CEEA™ instrument against the posterior wall of the stomach just above the crow's foot and adjacent to a #32F Ewald tube passed into the stomach and positioned along the lesser curvature. With the trocar tip, perforate the anterior and posterior walls of the stomach using the center of the anvil as a guide.

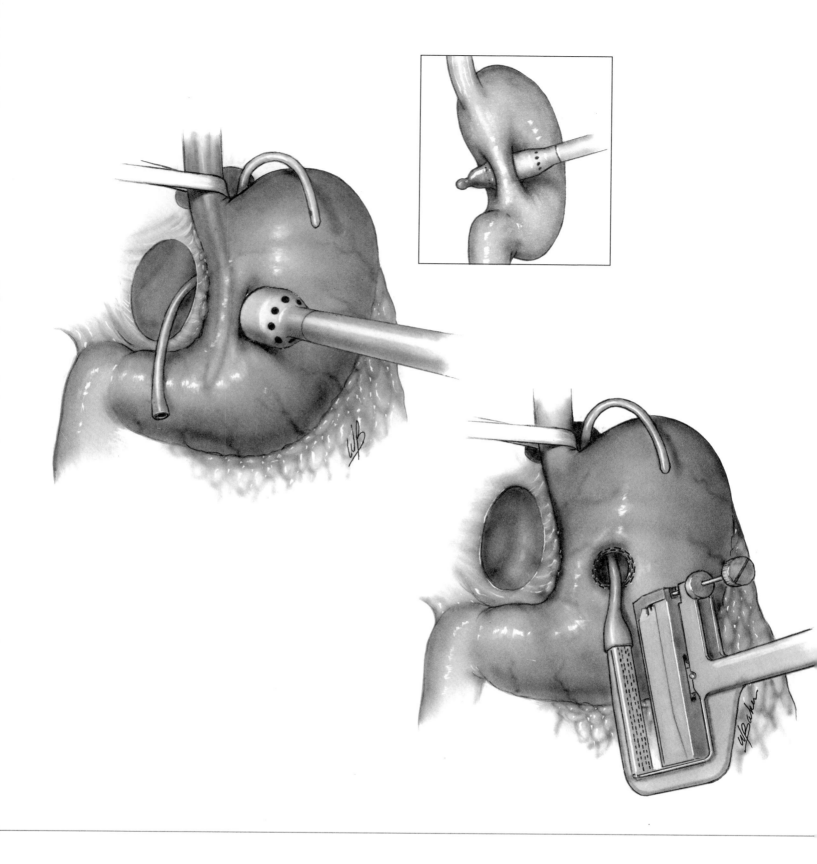

Advance the anvil shaft through the gastric opening. Remove the trocar tip and place the anvil on the anvil shaft. Close the instrument and fire the staples. A circular double staggered row of staples join the anterior and posterior walls of the stomach and the circular blade in the instrument cuts a window.

The vertical gastric partition is created using the TA 90 B™ instrument. Pass the flange end of the catheter through the window and attach it to the lower jaw of the TA 90 B™ instrument. Using the catheter as a guide, pass the lower jaw through the window and apply the instrument vertically across the stomach parallel to the lesser curvature.

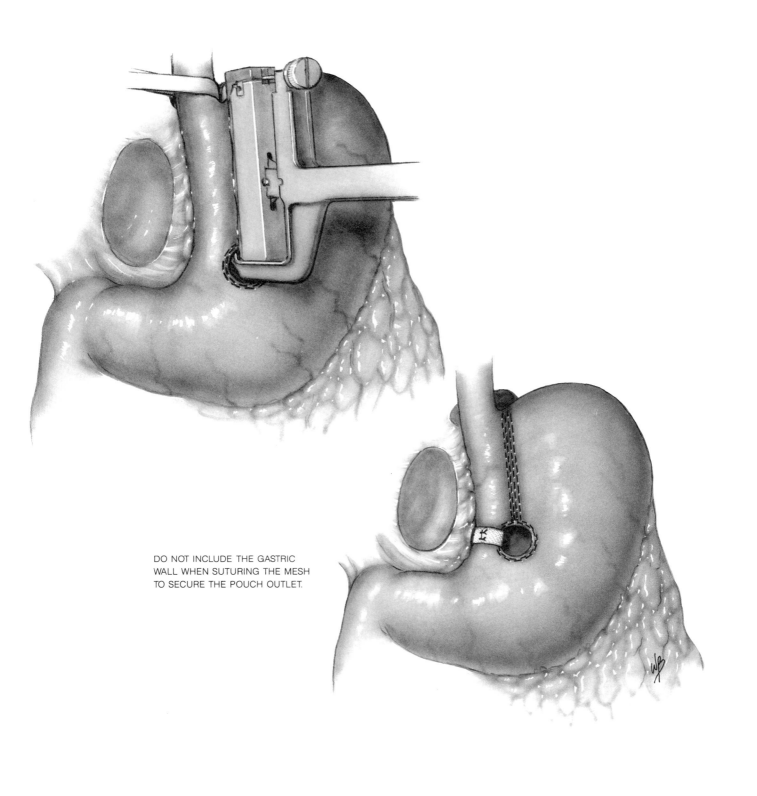

DO NOT INCLUDE THE GASTRIC
WALL WHEN SUTURING THE MESH
TO SECURE THE POUCH OUTLET.

Remove the catheter and screw the retaining pin firmly into place. Close the instrument, measure the pouch volume and fire the staples. Four parallel staggered rows of staples partition the stomach.

Mark a 7 x 1.5 cm. strip of polypropylene mesh at 5-5.5 cm. Wrap the mesh around the pouch outlet by passing an end through the window, posteriorly around the outlet and through an opening in the lesser omentum on the lesser curvature of the stomach. Secure the mesh to itself with three polypropylene sutures placed at the marking.

The greater omentum is sutured to the lesser omentum covering the gastric window and polypropylene band.

The fascia and skin are closed in the usual manner with the DFS™ instrument and the PREMIUM® skin stapler.

Silastic Ring
Vertical Gastroplasty

Auto Suture® Instruments Used in a
Silastic Ring Vertical Gastroplasty

See Cautions and Contraindications on page 236

INSTRUMENT	CLINICAL APPLICATION
TA 90 BN™ Instrument	Partition of the gastric pouch.
DFS™ Instrument and PREMIUM® Skin Stapler	Closure of fascia and skin.

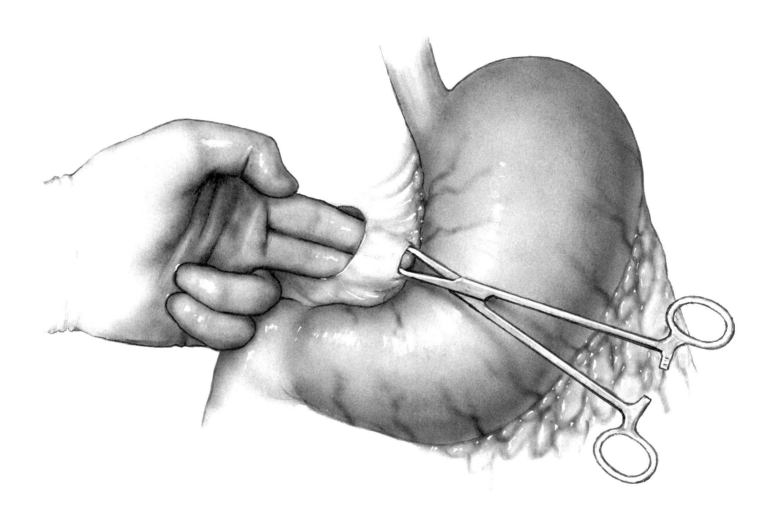

An opening is created in the lesser omentum adjacent
to the gastric wall and at the midpoint of the lesser
curvature.

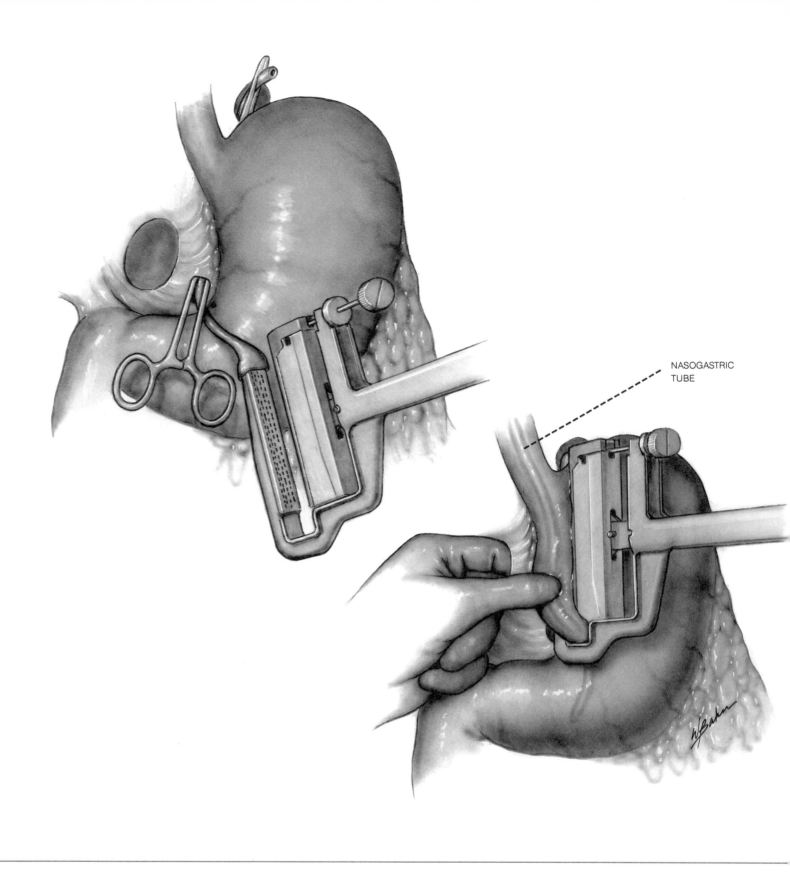

NASOGASTRIC
TUBE

A second opening is made in the gastrophrenic membrane 1-1.5 cm. left of the esophagus. A catheter is placed through the openings along the posterior wall of the stomach.

The TA 90 BN™ instrument is used to create a vertical partition of the gastric pouch. Attach the flange end of the catheter to the lower jaw of the instrument. Using the catheter as a guide, apply the TA 90 BN™ instrument vertically across the stomach from the lesser curvature to the esophagogastric junction. Remove the catheter and screw the retaining pin firmly into place. Close the instrument ensuring that the nasogastric tube and lesser curvature of the stomach are within the notch at the rear of the instrument. Measure the pouch volume and fire the staples.

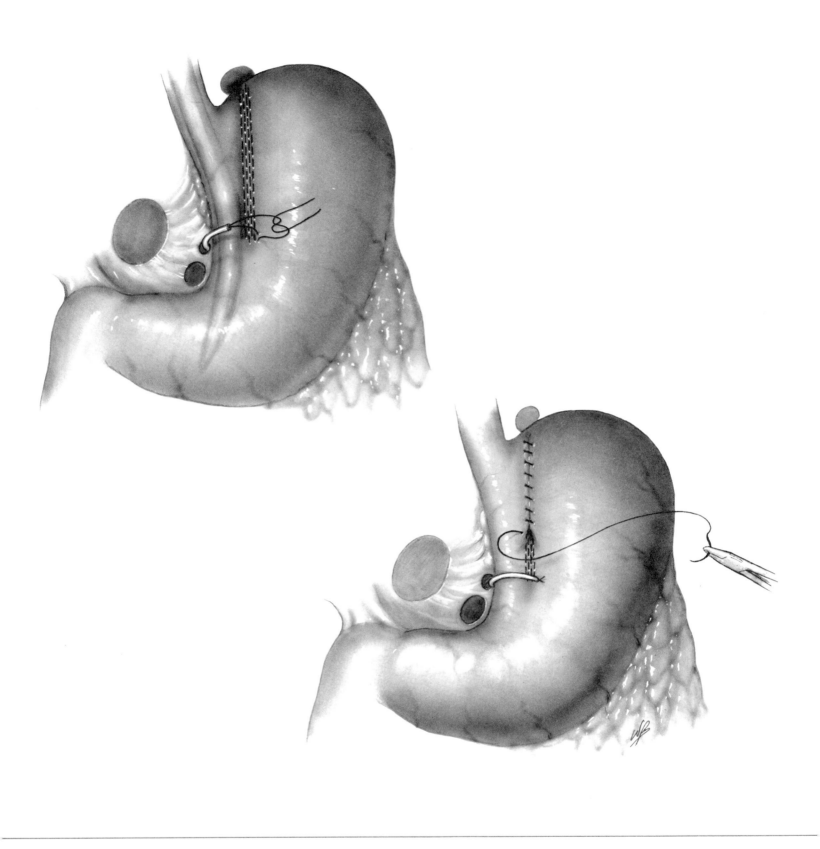

Four parallel staggered rows of staples partition the stomach leaving an outlet at the lesser curvature.

The nasogastric tube is replaced with a #32 Ewald tube and the pouch outlet is secured with a 42 mm. length of #10 silastic tubing and a 00 polypropylene suture. Tie the suture snugly so that the ring gently rests against the walls of the stomach.

The gastric staple line partition may be oversewn with a running suture.

The fascia and skin are closed in the usual manner with the DFS™ instrument and the PREMIUM® skin stapler.

Pyloroplasty

Auto Suture® Instruments Used in a Heineke-Mikulicz, Finney and Jaboulay Pyloroplasty

See Cautions and Contraindications on page 236

INSTRUMENT	CLINICAL APPLICATION
TA® 55 Instrument	Transverse closure of the longitudinal incision in a Heineke-Mikulicz Pyloroplasty. Closure of the stab wound in a Finney and Jaboulay Pyloroplasty. Alternate Technique: Closure of the gastrotomy in a Jaboulay Pyloroplasty.
GIA™ Instrument	Anastomosis of the duodenum to the antrum of the stomach in a Finney and Jaboulay Pyloroplasty.
EEA™ Instrument or PREMIUM CEEA™ Instrument	Alternate Technique: Anastomosis of the duodenum to the antrum of the stomach in a Jaboulay Pyloroplasty.
DFS™ Instrument and PREMIUM® Skin Stapler	Closure of fascia and skin.

Heineke-Mikulicz Pyloroplasty

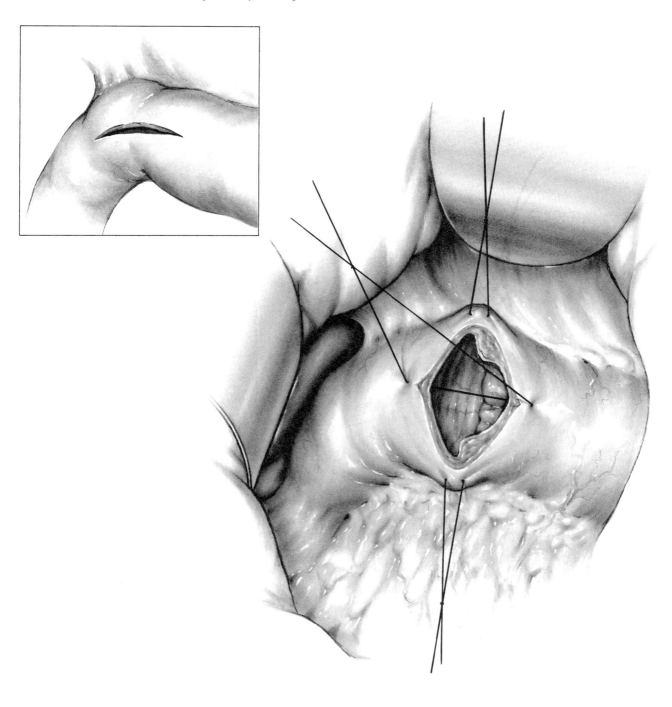

The usual longitudinal incision is made in the anterior wall of the duodenum and stomach across the pylorus. Place traction sutures at the midpoints of the incision and a single traction suture through the proximal and distal corners of the incision.

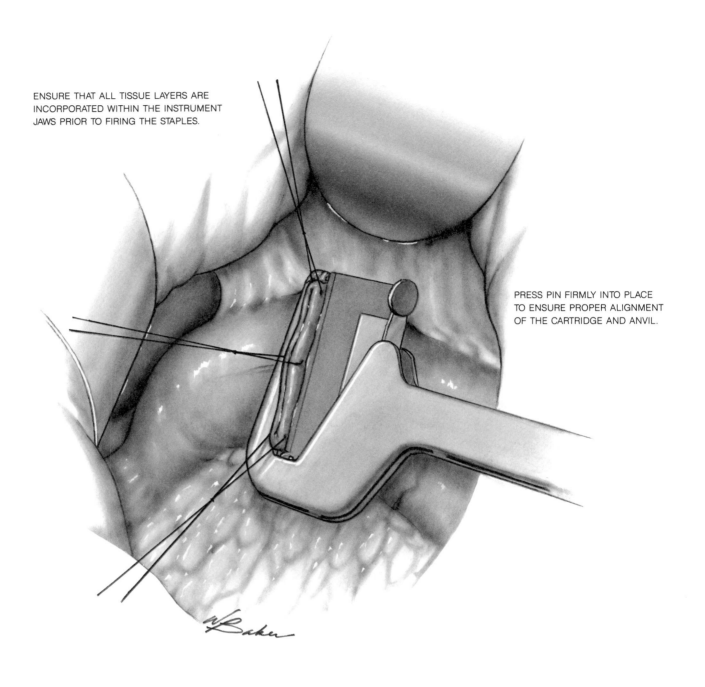

ENSURE THAT ALL TISSUE LAYERS ARE
INCORPORATED WITHIN THE INSTRUMENT
JAWS PRIOR TO FIRING THE STAPLES.

PRESS PIN FIRMLY INTO PLACE
TO ENSURE PROPER ALIGNMENT
OF THE CARTRIDGE AND ANVIL.

Convert the longitudinal incision to a transverse
closure by distracting the two midpoint sutures.

Slip the jaws of the TA® 55 instrument around the
tissue beneath the traction sutures, close the
instrument and fire the staples.

124

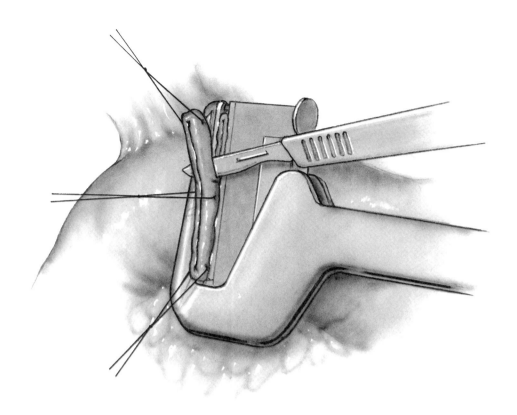

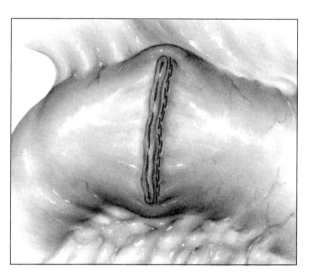

Before removing the instrument, use the TA® 55 instrument edge as a guide to excise the margin of tissue protruding through the jaws.

The tissue is joined with a double staggered row of staples.

Finney Pyloroplasty

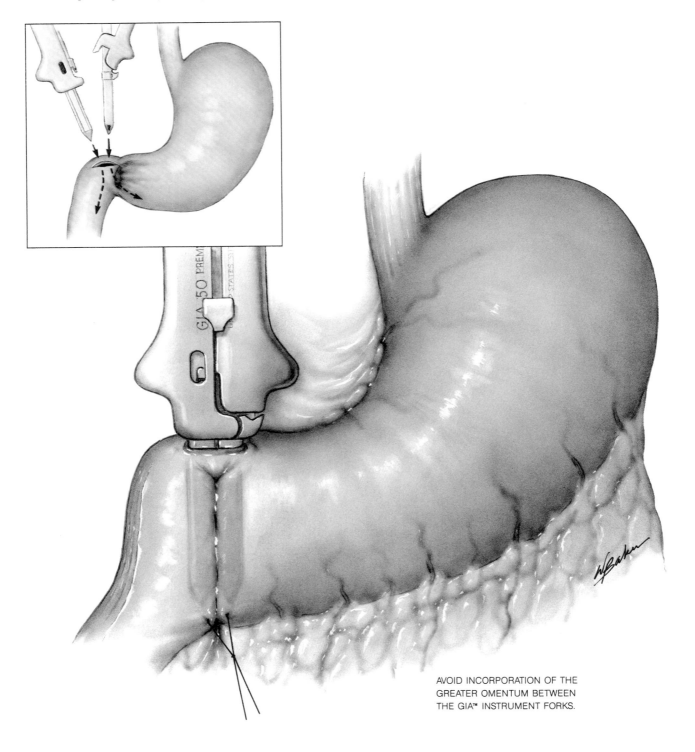

AVOID INCORPORATION OF THE
GREATER OMENTUM BETWEEN
THE GIA™ INSTRUMENT FORKS.

The usual Kocher mobilization of the duodenum is performed and a single traction suture is placed to approximate the greater curvature of the stomach to the inner margin of the duodenum, thus forming an inverted "U" with the pylorus at the apex.

The GIA™ instrument is used to perform the anastomosis. A 2 cm. longitudinal stab wound is made across the pylorus. Insert the cartridge fork of the instrument into the duodenum and the anvil fork into the antrum. Close the instrument and fire the staples. Two double staggered rows of staples join the duodenum and antrum; simultaneously, the knife blade in the instrument cuts between the two double staples lines.

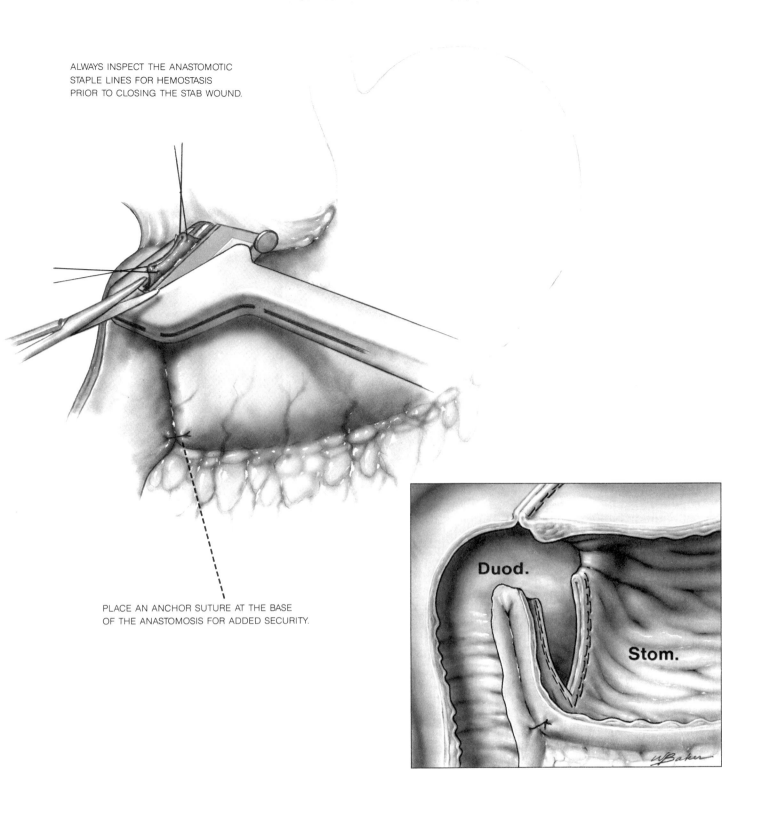

ALWAYS INSPECT THE ANASTOMOTIC
STAPLE LINES FOR HEMOSTASIS
PRIOR TO CLOSING THE STAB WOUND.

PLACE AN ANCHOR SUTURE AT THE BASE
OF THE ANASTOMOSIS FOR ADDED SECURITY.

Duod.

Stom.

The stab wound is closed transversely with the TA® 55
instrument.

Jaboulay Pyloroplasty

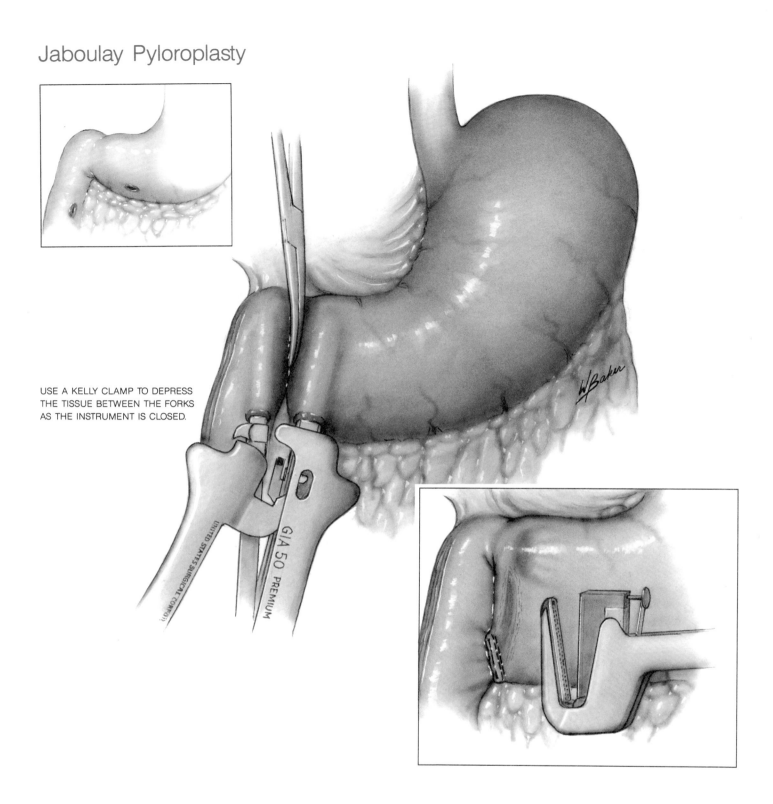

USE A KELLY CLAMP TO DEPRESS
THE TISSUE BETWEEN THE FORKS
AS THE INSTRUMENT IS CLOSED.

The usual Kocher mobilization of the duodenum is performed.

The GIA™ instrument is used to perform the gastro-duodenostomy. Corresponding stab wounds are made into the antrum of the stomach and the duodenum.

Insert one fork of the instrument into each lumen. Close the instrument and fire the staples. Inspect the anastomotic staple lines for hemostasis prior to transverse closure of the now common stab wound with the TA® 55 instrument.

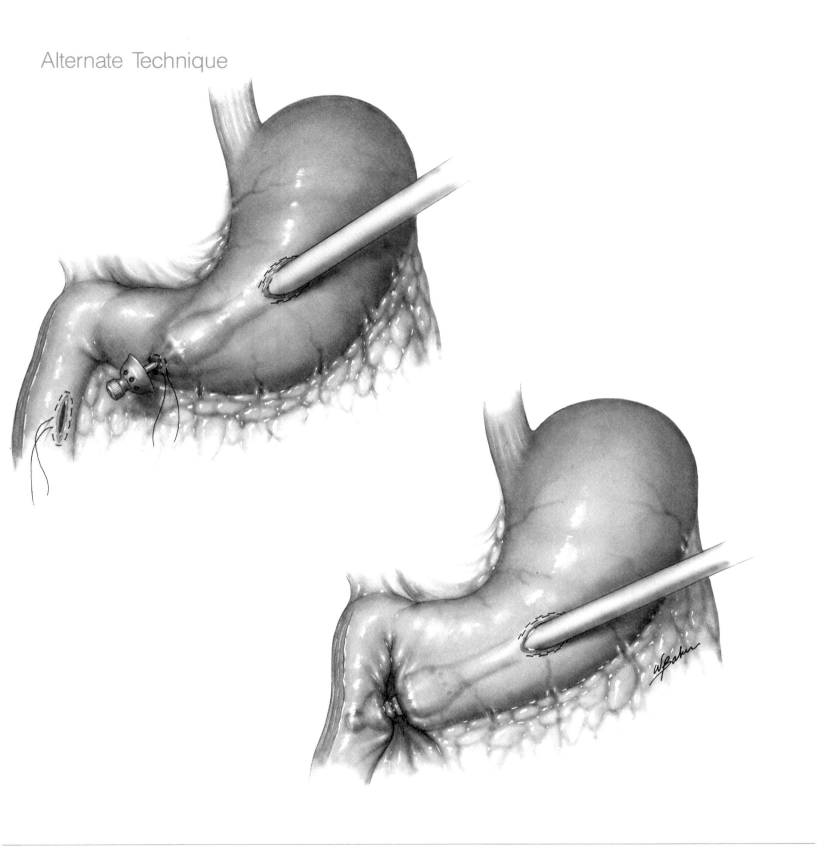

Alternate Technique

The gastroduodenostomy may be performed using the EEA™ instrument. Introduce the instrument, without anvil, through a gastrotomy. Incise the anterior wall of the antrum at the level of the anastomosis and place a manual purse string suture. Advance the center rod of the instrument through the opening and tie the purse string suture. Place the anvil on the center rod.

Make a 2.5-3 cm. corresponding incision into the lumen of the duodenum and place a manual purse string suture. Insert the anvil into the duodenum and tie the purse string suture. Close the instrument and fire the staples.

Inspect the anastomosis for hemostasis prior to closure of the gastrotomy with the TA® 55 instrument.

The fascia and skin are closed in the usual manner with the DFS™ instrument and the PREMIUM® skin stapler.

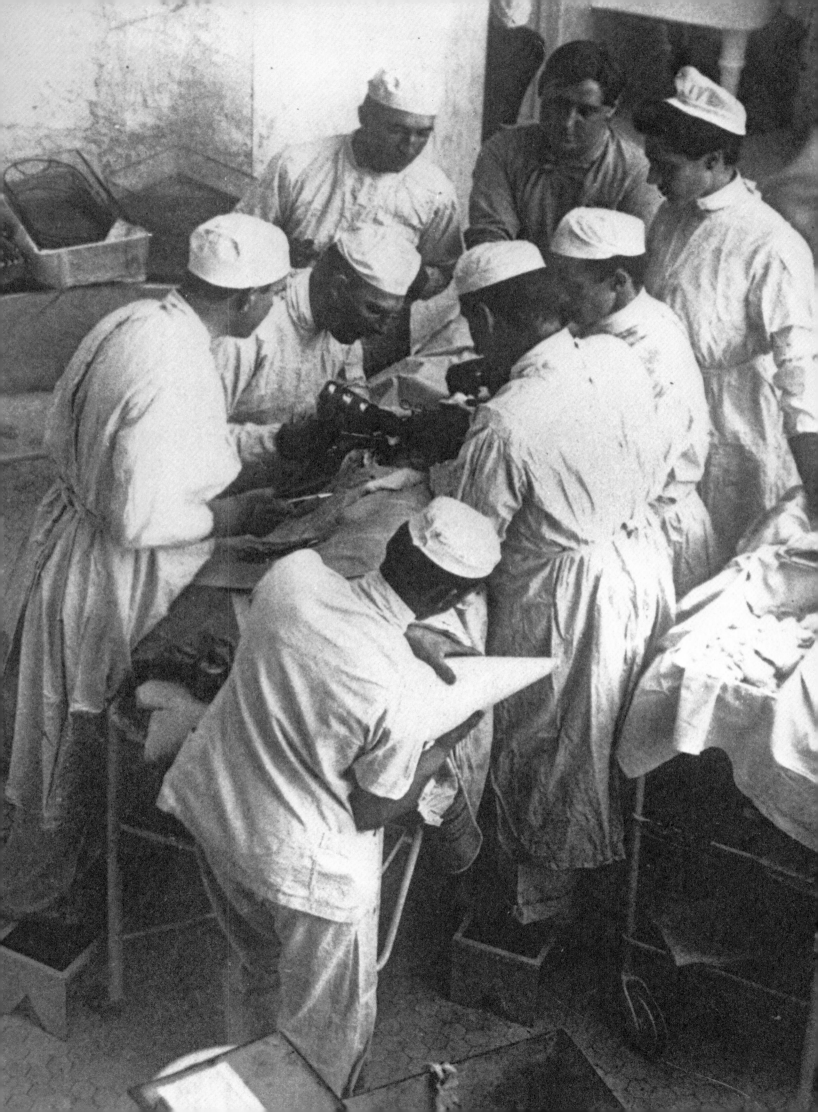

INTESTINAL SURGERY

ns Hopkins new amphitheater (1905).
ıped around operating table are
ʼoung, Dr. Halsted, Dr. Cushing,
inney.

End-to-End Anastomosis

Auto Suture® Instruments Used in an End-to-End Bowel Anastomosis

See Cautions and Contraindications on page 236

INSTRUMENT	CLINICAL APPLICATION
LDS™ Instrument	Ligation and division of the mesenteric vessels.
ROTICULATOR® 55 Instrument	Anastomosis of the proximal and distal large bowel.
TA® 55 Instrument	Anastomosis of the proximal and distal large bowel.
TA® 30 Instrument	Anastomosis of the proximal and distal small bowel.
DFS™ Instrument and PREMIUM® Skin Stapler	Closure of fascia and skin.

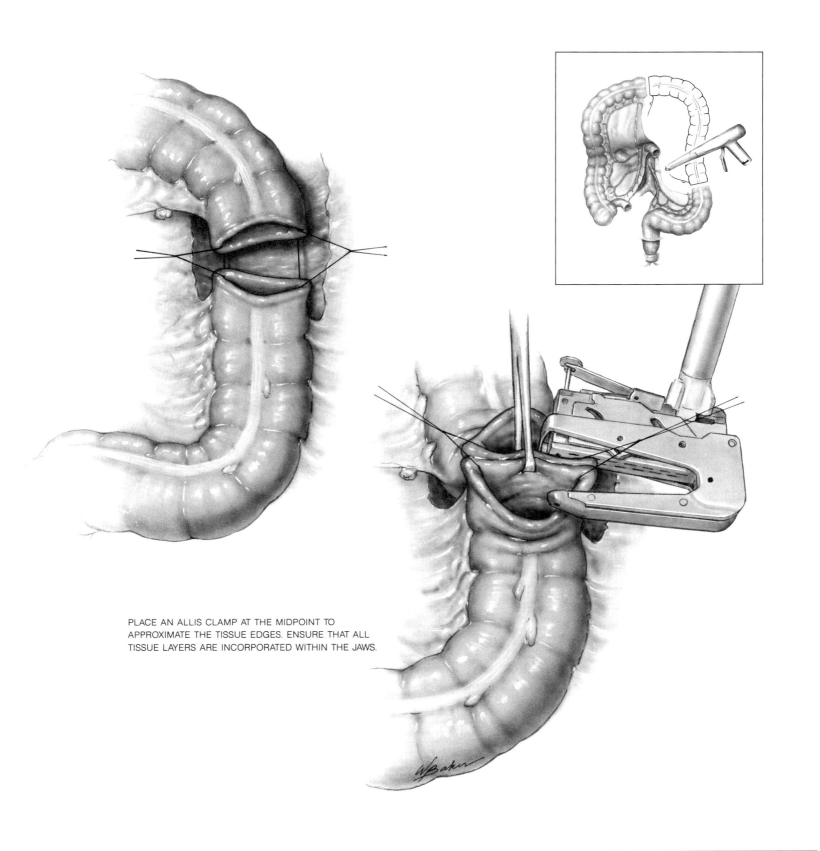

PLACE AN ALLIS CLAMP AT THE MIDPOINT TO
APPROXIMATE THE TISSUE EDGES. ENSURE THAT ALL
TISSUE LAYERS ARE INCORPORATED WITHIN THE JAWS.

The segment of bowel to be resected is mobilized
using the LDS™ instrument to ligate and divide the
mesenteric vessels. Slip the tissue to be ligated into
the jaw of the LDS™ instrument and fire the staples.
Two staples ligate the vessel; simultaneously, a knife
blade divides the vessel between the staples.

The bowel is resected in the usual manner.

The anastomosis is performed using the principle of
triangulation. Approximate the posterior walls of the
bowel with inverting traction sutures, serosa to serosa.
One traction suture aligns the mesenteric borders and
the second suture aligns the antimesenteric borders.
Slip the jaws of the ROTICULATOR® 55 instrument
around the tissue edges just beneath the traction
sutures.

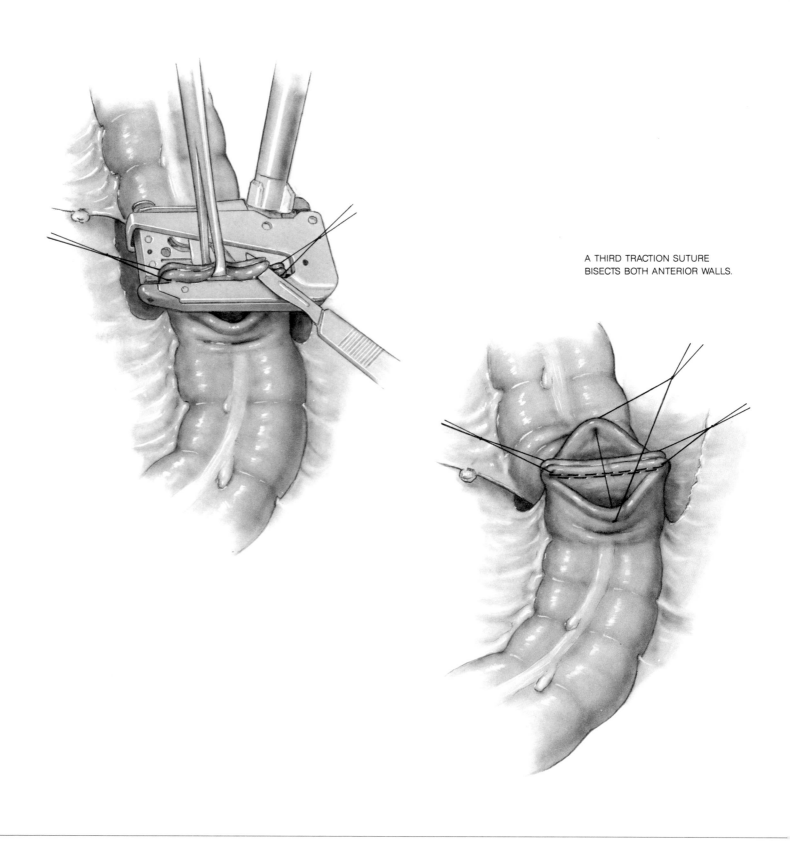

A THIRD TRACTION SUTURE
BISECTS BOTH ANTERIOR WALLS.

Close the instrument and fire the staples. Before removing the instrument and leaving the two traction sutures intact, excise the margin of tissue protruding through the jaws using the instrument edge as a cutting guide. The posterior wall forms the base of the triangle.

Bisect the anterior walls of the bowel with an everting traction suture.

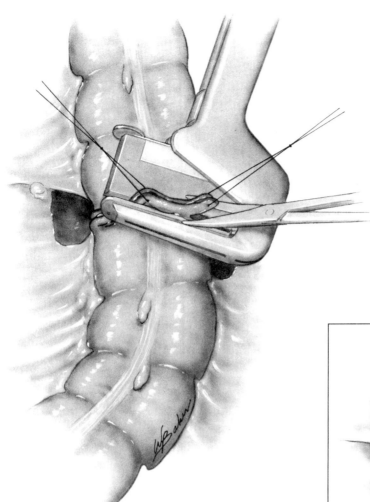

CARE MUST BE TAKEN TO OVERLAP THE
ENDS OF THE PREVIOUS STAPLE LINES.

THE TA® 30 INSTRUMENT MAY
BE USED DEPENDING ON THE
DIAMETER OF THE BOWEL.

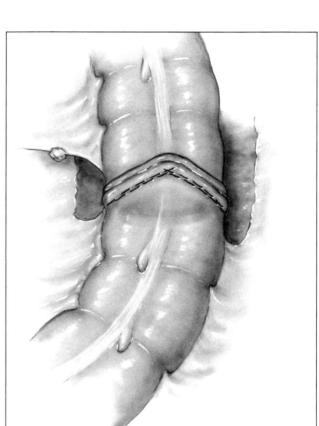

THE COMPLETED ANASTOMOSIS HAS ONE
INVERTED AND TWO EVERTED STAPLE LINES.

Each arm of the triangle is closed with one application of the TA® 55 instrument. Slip the jaws of the instrument around one side of the triangle. As the instrument is closed, make certain to include the end of the posterior staple line. Fire the staples. Before removing the instrument, excise the margin of tissue protruding through the jaws, leaving the apical traction suture intact.

Close the remaining side of the triangle in a similar fashion. Take care to include the end of the posterior staple line and the apex of the triangle to obtain a secure closure. This technique of anastomosis may be performed in a left hemicolectomy.

End-to-End Anastomosis
(for bowel that can be rotated)

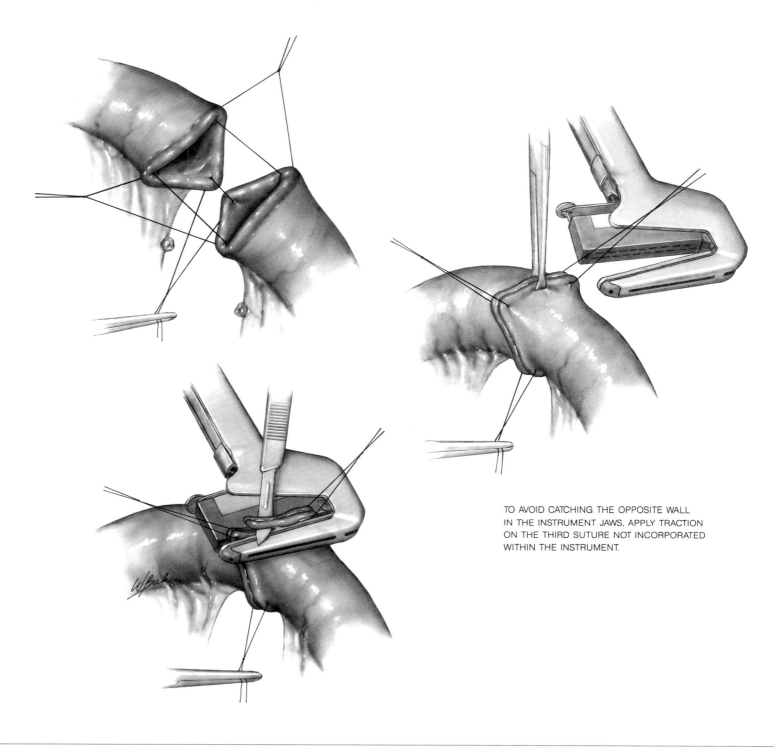

TO AVOID CATCHING THE OPPOSITE WALL
IN THE INSTRUMENT JAWS, APPLY TRACTION
ON THE THIRD SUTURE NOT INCORPORATED
WITHIN THE INSTRUMENT.

Using the principle of triangulation, the anastomosis is created with three applications of the TA® 30 instrument. Place three everting traction sutures equidistantly to approximate the bowel ends mucosa to mucosa. Align the mesenteric borders with the first traction suture and place the two remaining traction sutures at ⅓ intervals.

Slip the jaws of the TA® 30 instrument around the tissue just beneath the first two traction sutures. Close the instrument and fire the staples. Using the instrument edge as a guide, excise the margin of tissue protruding through the jaws, leaving the traction sutures intact.

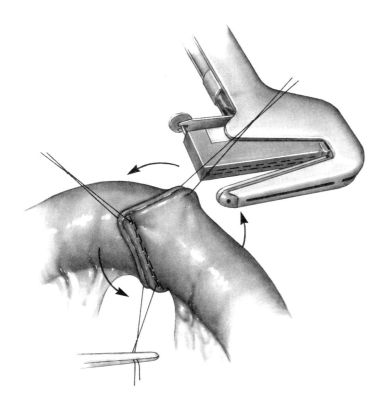

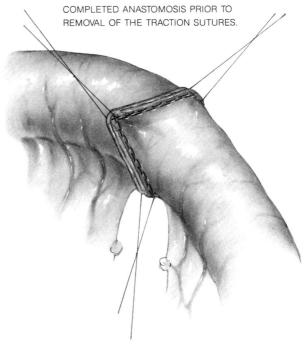

COMPLETED ANASTOMOSIS PRIOR TO
REMOVAL OF THE TRACTION SUTURES.

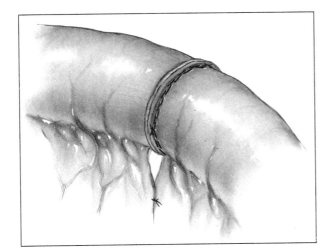

Repeat the procedure to close the second arm of the triangle. Take care to overlap the end of the previously placed staple line.

To bring the third arm of the triangle into position, rotate the bowel slightly and present the first traction suture through the rent in the mesentery. Reapply the

TA® 30 instrument, taking care to include the ends of the two previous staple lines.

The fascia and skin are closed in the usual manner with the DFS™ instrument and the PREMIUM® skin stapler.

Functional End-to-End Anastomosis

Auto Suture® Instruments Used in a Functional End-to-End Anastomosis

See Cautions and Contraindications on page 236

INSTRUMENT	CLINICAL APPLICATION
LDS™ Instrument	Ligation and division of the mesenteric vessels.
GIA™ Instrument	Closure and transection of the proximal and distal bowel. Anastomosis of the proximal and distal bowel.
TA® 55 Instrument	Closure of the common opening.
DFS™ Instrument and PREMIUM® Skin Stapler	Closure of fascia and skin.

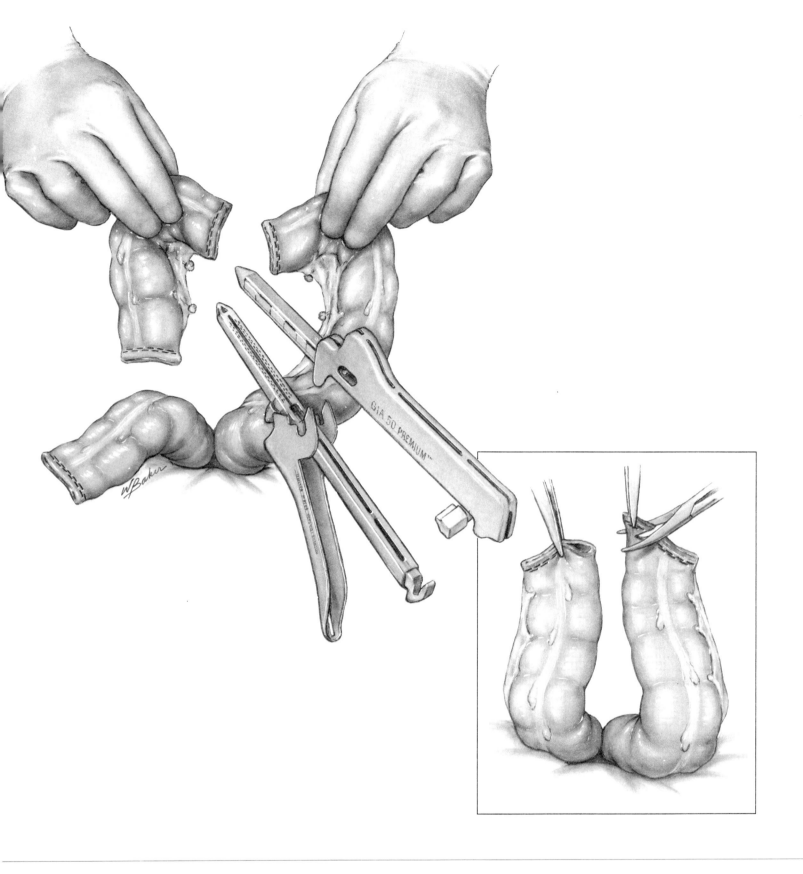

The segment of bowel to be resected is mobilized using the LDS™ instrument to ligate and divide the mesenteric vessels.

The bowel resection is performed with two applications of the GIA™ instrument. Place the instrument around the bowel at the point of transection in a scissor-like fashion. Close the instrument and fire the staples. A double staggered staple line is placed on the patient side and a second double staggered staple line is placed on the specimen side; simultaneously, a knife blade in the instrument transects the bowel between the two double staple lines. Reapply the GIA™ instrument and resect the specimen. The bowel is closed prior to resection, reducing the possibility of intraperitoneal contamination.

The GIA™ instrument is used to perform the entero-enterostomy. Excise the antimesenteric corner of the staple line closure of both the proximal and distal bowel.

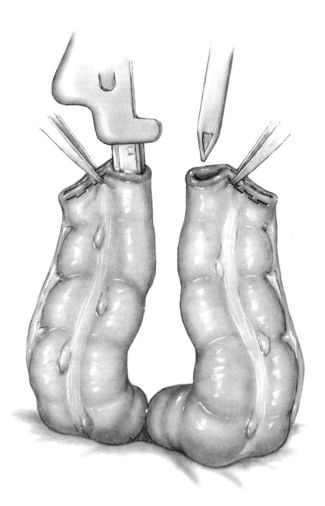

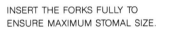
INSERT THE FORKS FULLY TO
ENSURE MAXIMUM STOMAL SIZE.

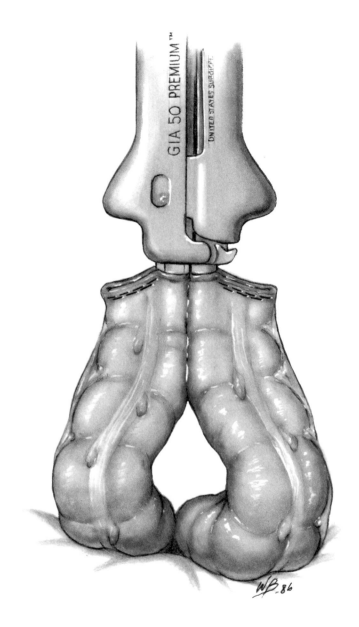

Approximate the antimesenteric borders of the proximal and distal bowel and insert one fork of the GIA™ instrument into each bowel lumen.

Align the bowel ends evenly on the instrument forks.

Close the instrument and fire the staples. Two double staggered staple lines join the bowel; simultaneously, the knife blade divides between the two double staple lines creating a stoma. Remove the instrument and inspect the anastomotic staple lines for hemostasis.

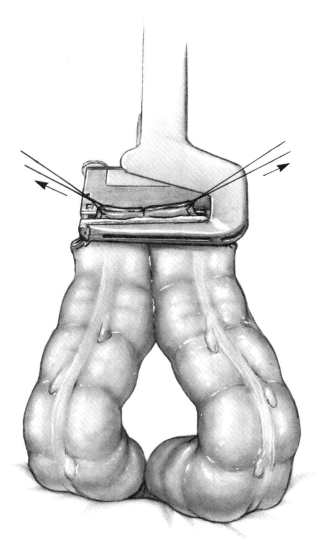

CARE MUST BE TAKEN TO OVERLAP THE ENDS OF THE PREVIOUS STAPLE LINES.

AVOID DIRECT APPOSITION OF THE ANASTOMOTIC STAPLE LINES.

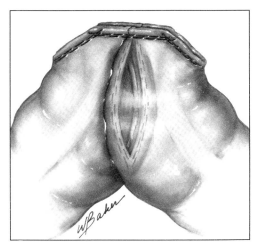

AN ANCHOR SUTURE MAY BE PLACED AT THE BASE OF THE ANASTOMOSIS FOR ADDITIONAL SECURITY.

The TA® 55 instrument is used to close the now common opening. Place an everting traction suture around each transection staple line and hold the sutures in opposition. A third traction suture or Allis clamp may be used at the midpoint. Place the jaws of the instrument around the tissue beneath the traction sutures. As the instrument is closed, make sure that the end of all previously placed staple lines and all tissue layers are incorporated within the jaws of the TA® 55 instrument. Fire the staples and prior to removal of the instrument, excise the redundant tissue using the instrument edge as a cutting guide.

Offset Anastomosis

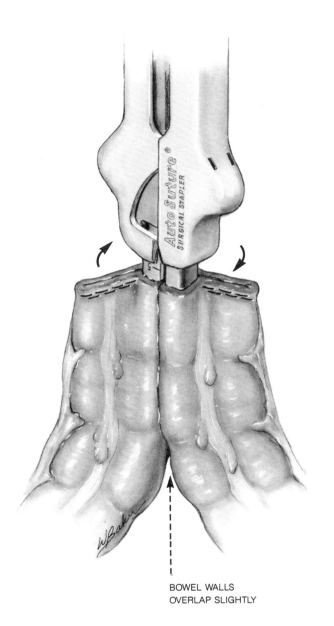

BOWEL WALLS
OVERLAP SLIGHTLY

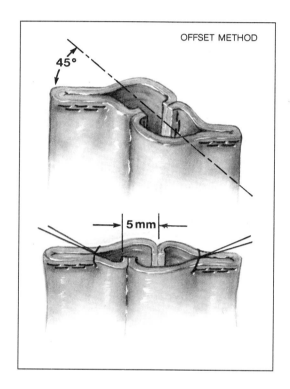

OFFSET METHOD

45°

5 mm

The bowel is mobilized and resected as previously described.

The GIA™ instrument is used to perform the anastomosis. Excise the antimesenteric corner of each

staple line closure. Insert one fork of the instrument into each bowel lumen. Rotate the instrument 45° relative to the transection staple lines. Alternately, the instrument can be held in place and the bowel rotated. Close the instrument and fire the staples.

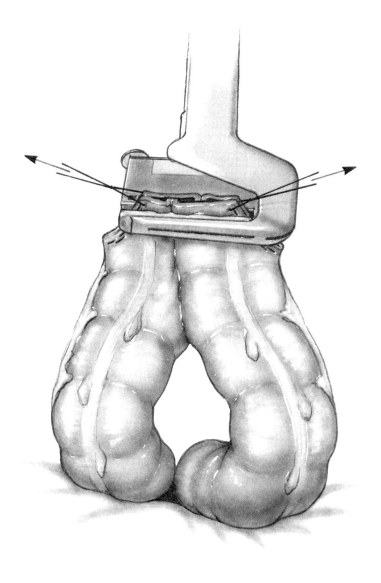

CARE MUST BE TAKEN TO OVERLAP THE
ENDS OF THE PREVIOUS STAPLE LINES.

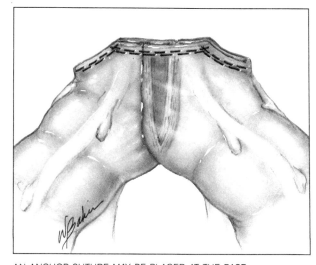

AN ANCHOR SUTURE MAY BE PLACED AT THE BASE
OF THE ANASTOMOSIS FOR ADDITIONAL SECURITY.

Inspect the anastomotic staple lines for hemostasis
prior to closure of the now common opening with
the TA® 55 instrument.

The resulting anastomosis is illustrated with the anterior
wall made transparent to depict the reconstruction.

143

Open Lumina Technique

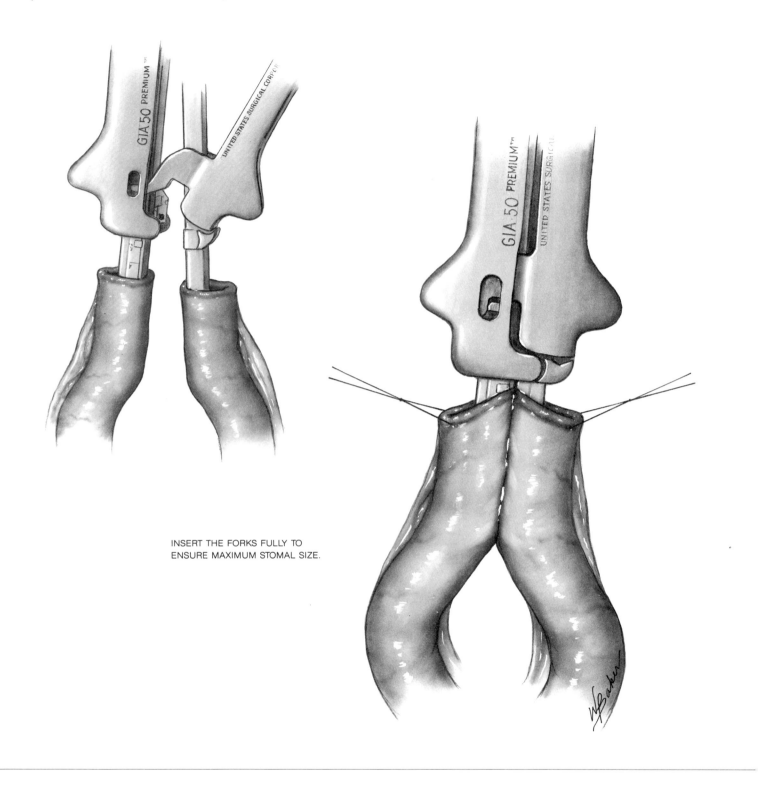

INSERT THE FORKS FULLY TO
ENSURE MAXIMUM STOMAL SIZE.

The bowel is mobilized using the LDS™ instrument and the specimen is resected manually in the usual manner.

The GIA™ instrument is used to perform the anastomosis. Approximate the antimesenteric borders of the bowel and insert one fork of the instrument into each lumen.

Align the bowel ends evenly on the forks, close the instrument and fire the staples. Two double staggered staple lines join the bowel; simultaneously, the knife blade divides between the two double staple lines creating a stoma.

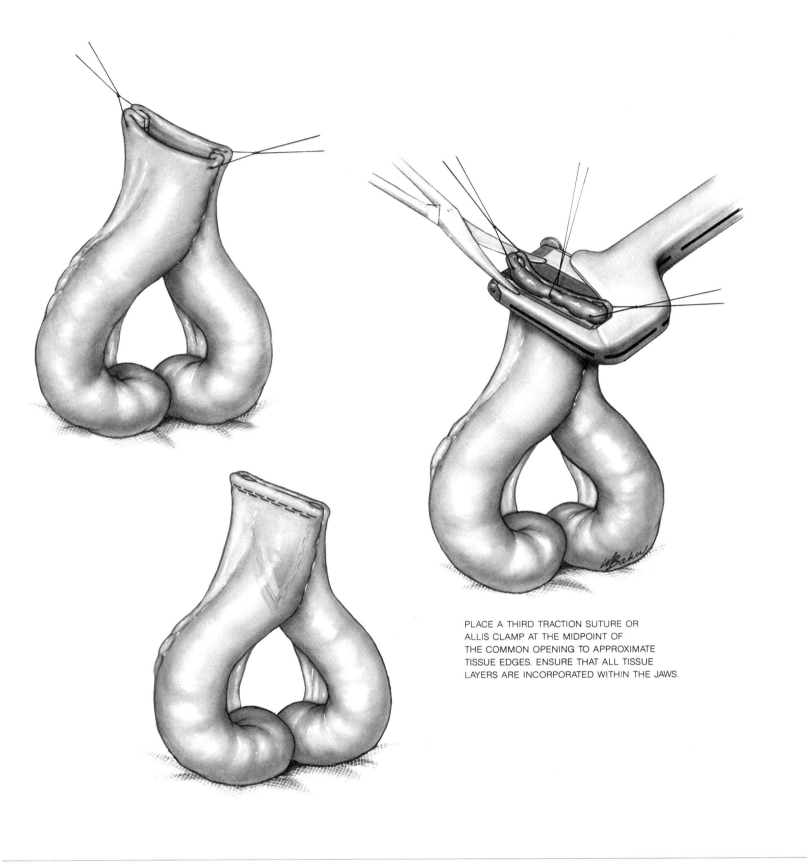

PLACE A THIRD TRACTION SUTURE OR
ALLIS CLAMP AT THE MIDPOINT OF
THE COMMON OPENING TO APPROXIMATE
TISSUE EDGES. ENSURE THAT ALL TISSUE
LAYERS ARE INCORPORATED WITHIN THE JAWS.

Inspect the anastomosis for hemostasis prior to closure of the common opening. Place an everting traction suture around each anastomotic staple line and distract the sutures. The wound edges are approximated in an everted manner with the anastomotic staple lines held apart and the stoma held open. Slip the jaws of the TA® 55 instrument around the tissue, close the instrument and fire the staples. Prior to removal, use the instrument edge as a guide to excise the margin of tissue protruding through the jaws.

One Stage Functional End-to-End Anastomosis and Resection

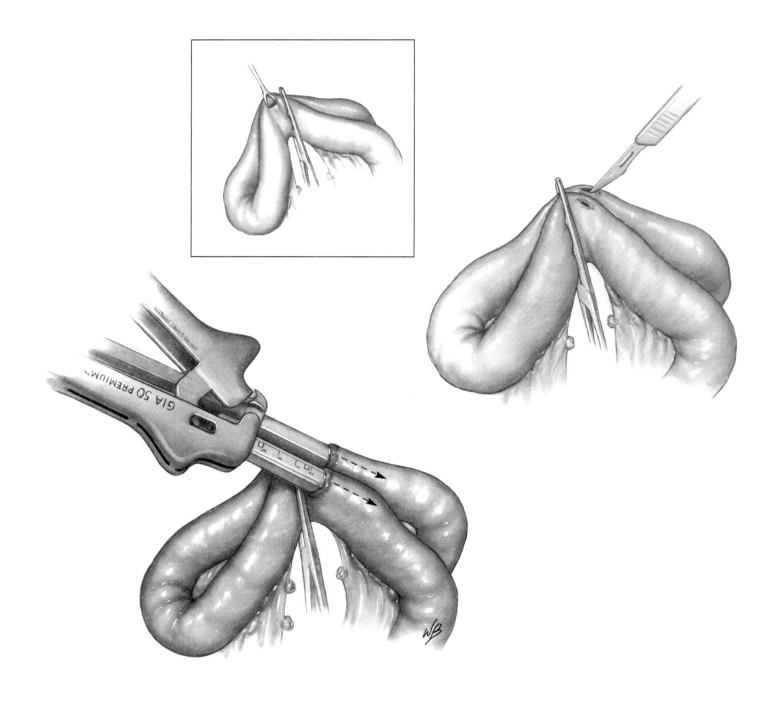

Following mobilization, the enteroenterostomy is performed using the GIA™ instrument. Loop the portion of bowel to be resected and approximate the antimesenteric borders with a Babcock clamp. Place a Kocher clamp at a 60° angle across both bowel at the transition between viable and nonviable intestine. Make a 1 cm. stab wound into the lumen of both the proximal and distal limbs.

Insert one fork of the GIA™ instrument into each lumen, close the instrument and fire the staples. Two double staggered rows of staples join the bowel; simultaneously, the knife blade cuts between the two double staple lines creating a stoma. Inspect the anastomotic staple lines for hemostasis.

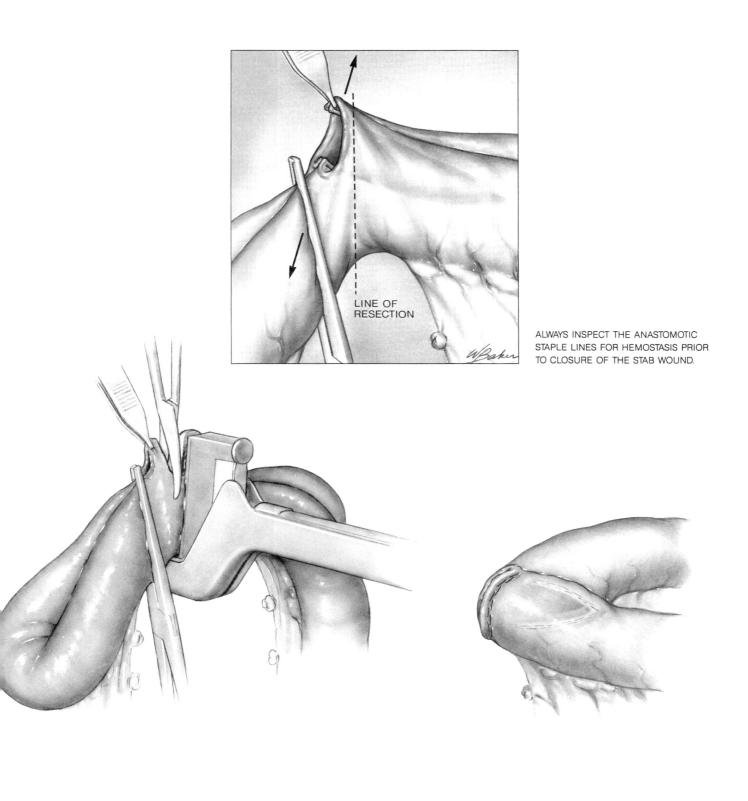

LINE OF
RESECTION

ALWAYS INSPECT THE ANASTOMOTIC
STAPLE LINES FOR HEMOSTASIS PRIOR
TO CLOSURE OF THE STAB WOUND.

The end of the anterior anastomotic staple line is grasped with forceps or an Allis clamp holding the anastomotic staple lines in opposition and the stoma open.

Slip the jaws of the TA® 55 instrument around both the proximal and distal bowel. Close the instrument and fire the staples. Prior to removing the instrument,

resect the specimen using the instrument edge as a cutting guide. The resulting anastomosis is illustrated with the bowel wall made transparent to depict the reconstruction.

The fascia and skin are closed in the usual manner with the DFS™ instrument and the PREMIUM® skin stapler.

Bypass Enteroenterostomy

Auto Suture® Instruments Used in a Bypass Enteroenterostomy

See Cautions and Contraindications on page 236

INSTRUMENT	CLINICAL APPLICATION
GIA™ Instrument	Anastomosis of the bowel loops.
TA® 55 Instrument	Closure of the common stab wound.
DFS™ Instrument and PREMIUM® Skin Stapler	Closure of fascia and skin.

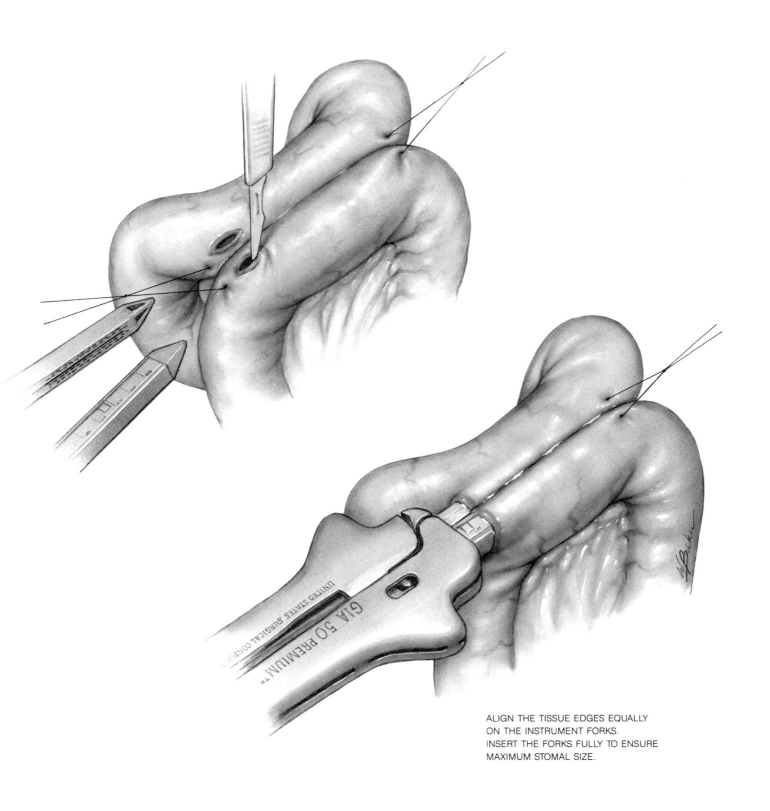

ALIGN THE TISSUE EDGES EQUALLY
ON THE INSTRUMENT FORKS.
INSERT THE FORKS FULLY TO ENSURE
MAXIMUM STOMAL SIZE.

The enteroenterostomy is performed with the GIA™ instrument. Using traction sutures, approximate the antimesenteric borders of the bowel to be anastomosed in a side-to-side fashion. Make a 1 cm. stab wound into the lumen of each bowel segment and insert one fork of the instrument into each lumen. Close the instrument and fire the staples.

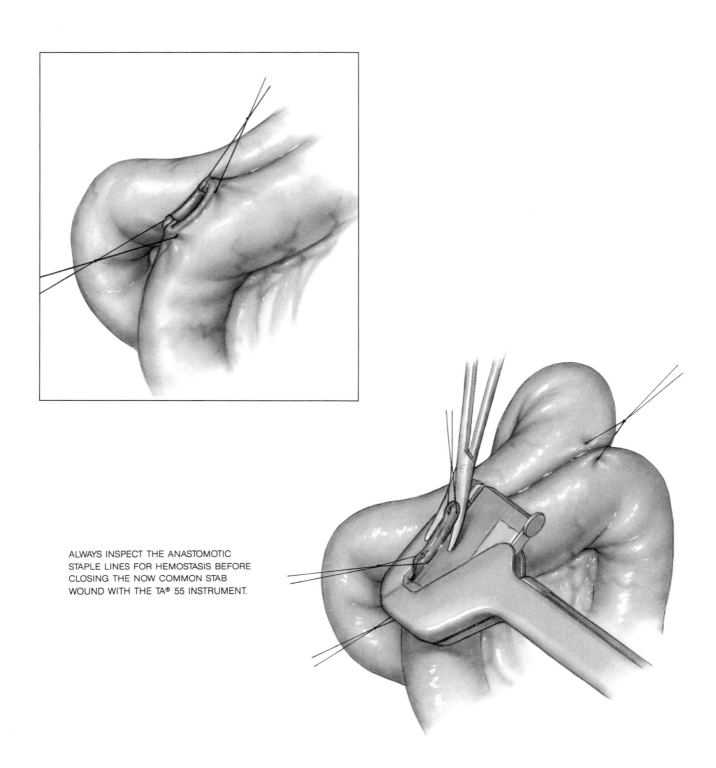

ALWAYS INSPECT THE ANASTOMOTIC
STAPLE LINES FOR HEMOSTASIS BEFORE
CLOSING THE NOW COMMON STAB
WOUND WITH THE TA® 55 INSTRUMENT.

Place an everting traction suture around each anastomotic staple line and distract the sutures, thus approximating the wound edges in an everted manner with the stoma held open. Slip the jaws of the TA® 55 instrument around the tissue just beneath the traction sutures. Close the instrument and fire the staples. Prior to removing the instrument, use the instrument edge as a guide to excise the margin of tissue protruding through the jaws.

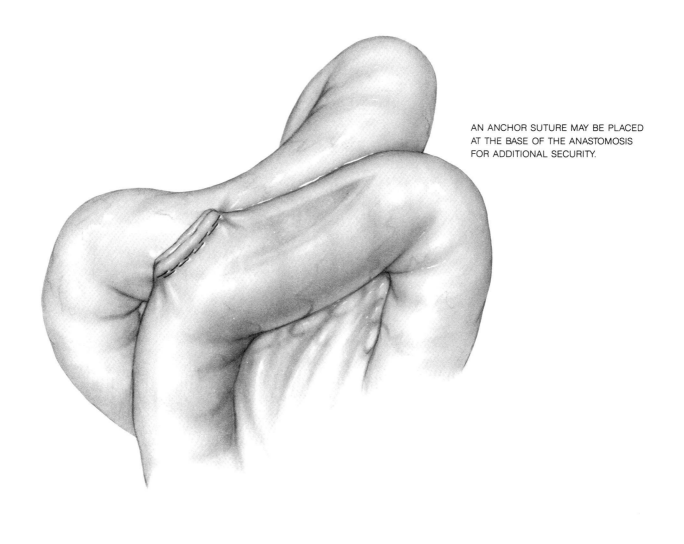

AN ANCHOR SUTURE MAY BE PLACED
AT THE BASE OF THE ANASTOMOSIS
FOR ADDITIONAL SECURITY.

The enteroenterostomy is illustrated with the anterior wall made transparent to depict the reconstruction.

The fascia and skin are closed in the usual manner with the DFS™ instrument and the PREMIUM® skin stapler.

Diverticulectomy

Auto Suture® Instruments Used in a Diverticulectomy

See Cautions and Contraindications on page 236

INSTRUMENT	CLINICAL APPLICATION
TA® 30 Instrument or TA® 55 Instrument	Closure of the base of the diverticulum.
DFS™ Instrument and PREMIUM® Skin Stapler	Closure of fascia and skin.

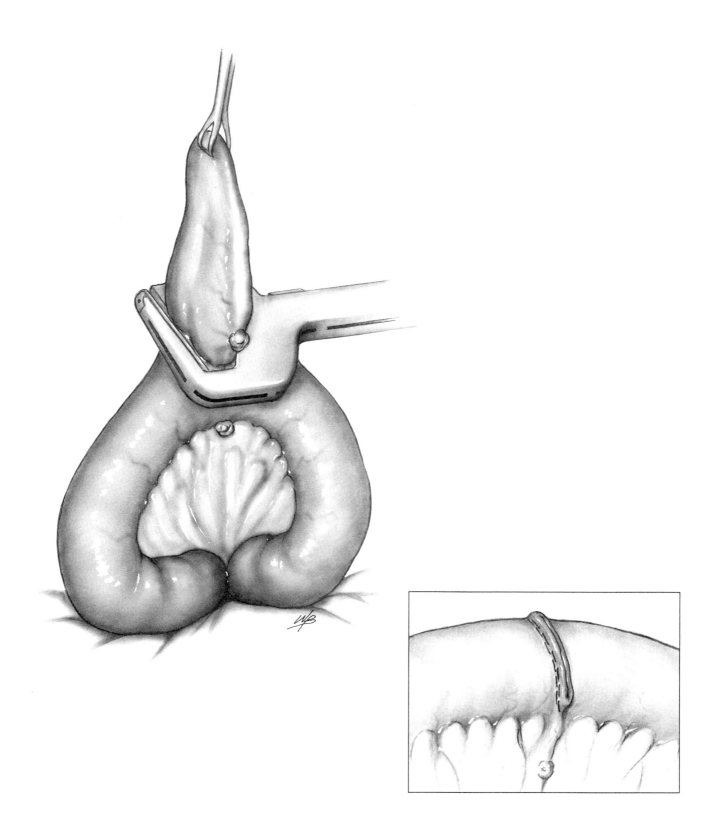

Any mesenteric vessel to the diverticulum should be ligated and divided.

The TA® 30 instrument or TA® 55 instrument is used to perform the diverticulectomy. Slip the jaws of the instrument around the base of the diverticulum. Close the instrument and fire the staples. Prior to removing the instrument, resect the diverticulum using the instrument edge as a cutting guide.

The fascia and skin are closed in the usual manner with the DFS™ instrument and the PREMIUM® skin stapler.

Appendectomy

Auto Suture® Instruments Used in an Appendectomy

See Cautions and Contraindications on page 236

INSTRUMENT	CLINICAL APPLICATION
TA® 30 Instrument	Closure of the base of the appendix.
GIA™ Instrument	Alternate technique: Closure of the base of the appendix.
DFS™ Instrument and PREMIUM® Skin Stapler	Closure of fascia and skin.

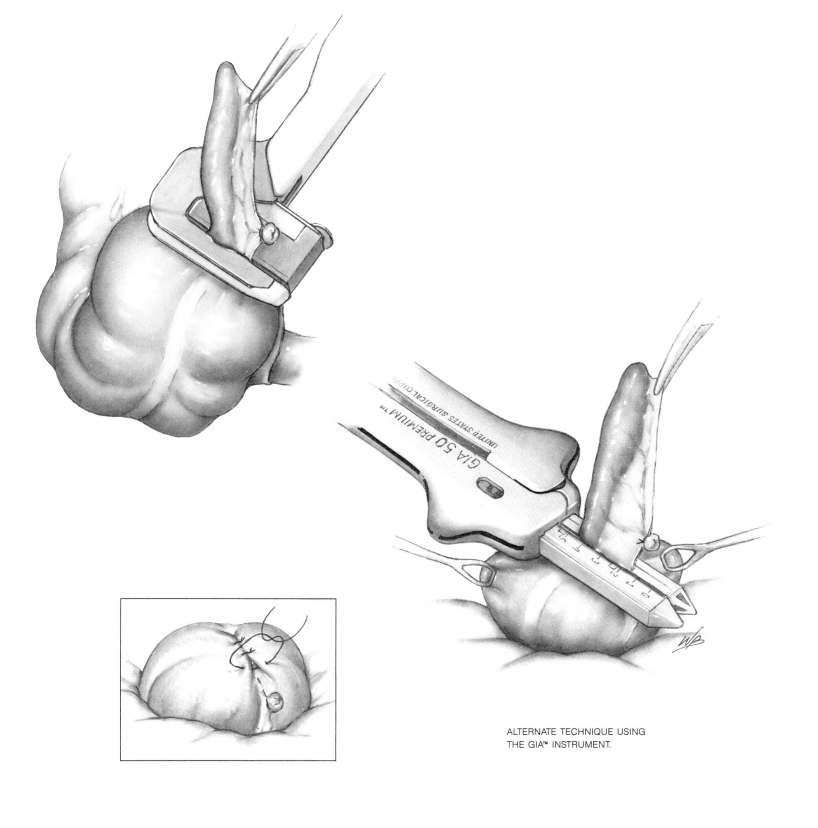

ALTERNATE TECHNIQUE USING
THE GIA™ INSTRUMENT.

The TA® 30 instrument may be used to perform the appendectomy. Slip the jaws of the instrument around the tissue at the appendicocecal junction, close the instrument and fire the staples. Before removing the instrument, use the instrument edge as a guide to resect the appendix. The cecal cuff is inverted with interrupted Lembert sutures.

As an alternate technique, the appendectomy may be performed with the GIA™ instrument. Place the instrument around the tissue at the appendicocecal junction, close the instrument and fire the staples. A double staggered staple line is placed on the cecum and a second double staggered staple line on the appendix; simultaneously, a knife blade resects the appendix between the two double staple lines.

The fascia and skin are closed in the usual manner with the DFS™ instrument and the PREMIUM® skin stapler.

Resection of Terminal Ileum and Ileocecostomy

Auto Suture® Instruments Used in
Resection of Terminal Ileum and Ileocecostomy with Incidental Appendectomy

See Cautions and Contraindications on page 236

INSTRUMENT	CLINICAL APPLICATION
LDS™ Instrument	Ligation and division of the mesenteric vessels.
GIA™ Instrument	Closure and transection of the proximal and distal ileum. Anastomosis of the ileum to the cecum.
TA® 55 Instrument	Closure of the common opening and base of the appendix.
DFS™ Instrument and PREMIUM® Skin Stapler	Closure of fascia and skin.

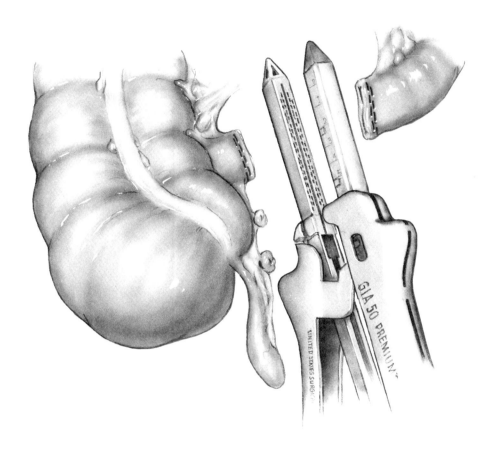

The appendix and ileum to be resected are mobilized using the LDS™ instrument to ligate and divide the mesenteric vessels.

The ileum is resected between two applications of the GIA™ instrument. Place the instrument around the ileum at the point of transection. Close the instrument and fire the staples. Two double staggered staple lines seal the ileum; simultaneously, a knife blade in the instrument transects the ileum between the two double staple lines. Reapply the instrument to complete the resection.

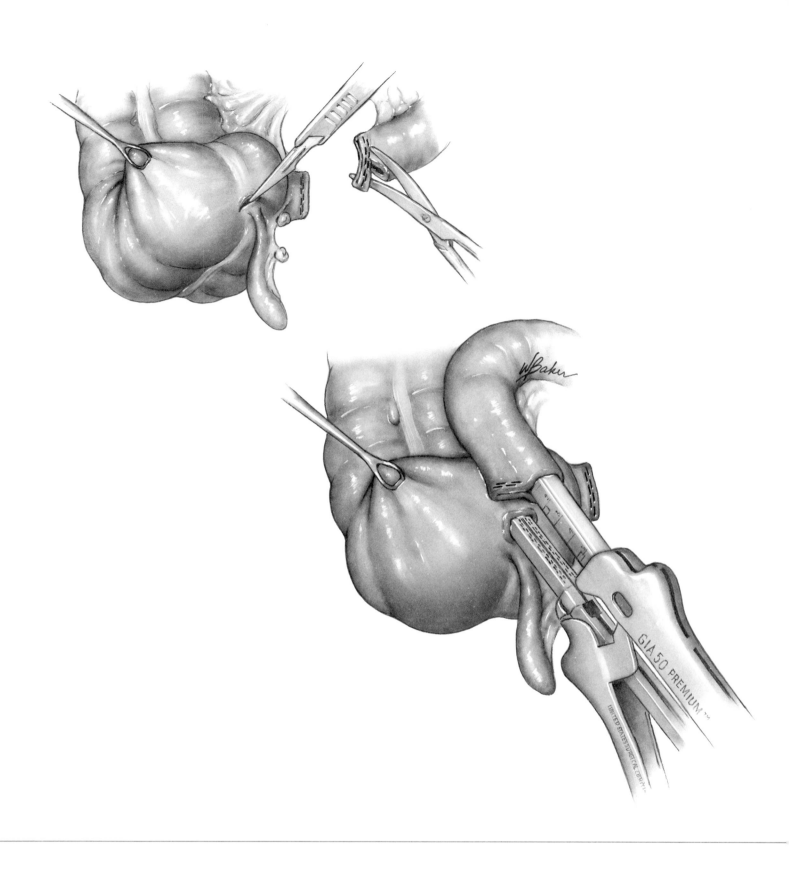

The GIA™ instrument is used to perform the ileocecostomy. Excise the antimesenteric corner of the staple line closure of the proximal ileum. Make a 1 cm. stab wound into the lumen of the cecum just above the appendix. Insert one fork of the GIA™ instrument into each lumen. Close the instrument and fire the staples. Remove the instrument and inspect the anastomotic staple lines for hemostasis.

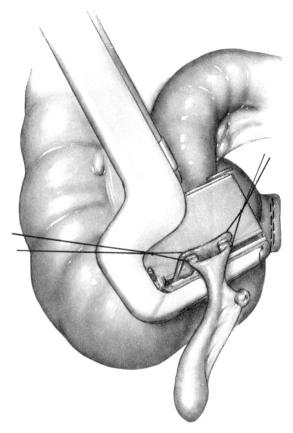

CARE MUST BE TAKEN TO OVERLAP THE
ENDS OF THE PREVIOUS STAPLE LINES.

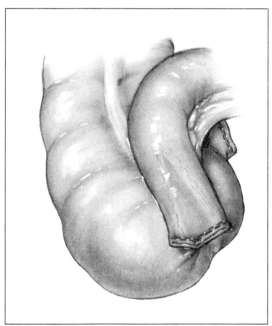

The TA® 55 instrument is used to close the now common opening and the base of the appendix. Place an everting traction suture around each anastomotic staple line and hold the staple lines in opposition. Slip the jaws of the TA® 55 instrument around the tissue beneath the traction sutures and appendix. Close the

instrument, fire the staples and resect the tissue using the instrument edge as a cutting guide prior to removing the instrument.

The fascia and skin are closed in the usual manner with the DFS™ instrument and the PREMIUM® skin stapler.

Bypass Ileocolostomy

Auto Suture® Instruments Used in a
Bypass Ileocolostomy

See Cautions and Contraindications on page 236

INSTRUMENT	CLINICAL APPLICATION
GIA™ Instrument	Anastomosis of the ileum to the colon.
TA® 55 Instrument	Closure of the common stab wound.
EEA™ Instrument or PREMIUM CEEA™ Instrument	Alternate technique: Anastomosis of the ileum to the colon.
TA® 30 Instrument	Alternate technique: Closure of the ileotomy.
DFS™ Instrument and PREMIUM® Skin Stapler	Closure of fascia and skin.

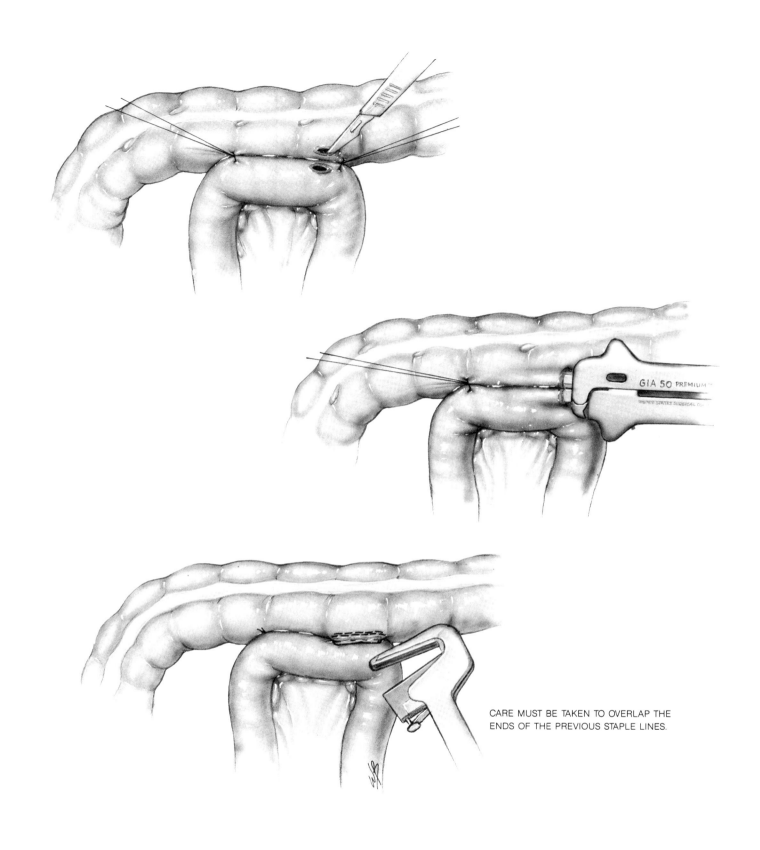

CARE MUST BE TAKEN TO OVERLAP THE
ENDS OF THE PREVIOUS STAPLE LINES.

The ileocolostomy is performed with the GIA™ instrument. Using two traction sutures, approximate the antimesenteric borders of the ileum and colon to be anastomosed. Make a 1 cm. stab wound into the lumen of each segment. Insert one fork of the GIA™ instrument into each lumen. Close the instrument and fire the staples. Inspect the anastomotic staple lines for hemostasis prior to closing the now common stab wound with the TA® 55 instrument.

Alternate Technique

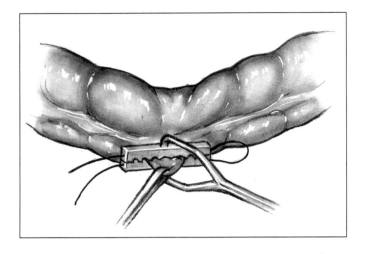

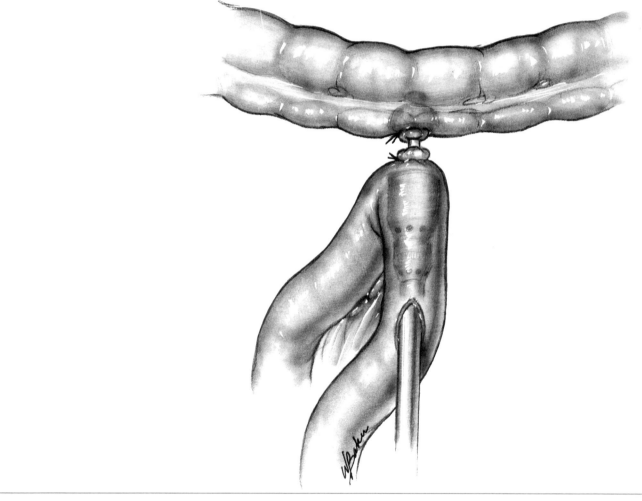

Identify the site of anastomosis of the ileum and colon. Grasp the antimesocolic border of the colon with an Allis clamp. Apply the purse string instrument just beneath the Allis clamp and place a purse string suture. Excise the excess tissue using the purse string instrument as a cutting guide.

The EEA™ instrument, without anvil, is introduced through a proximal ileotomy. The center rod is advanced

through an antimesenteric stab wound surrounded by a purse string suture. Tie the purse string suture and place the anvil on the center rod.

Remove the purse string instrument and introduce the anvil into the lumen of the colon. The use of three Allis clamps or three traction sutures on the colotomy edges facilitates insertion of the anvil. Tie the purse string suture.

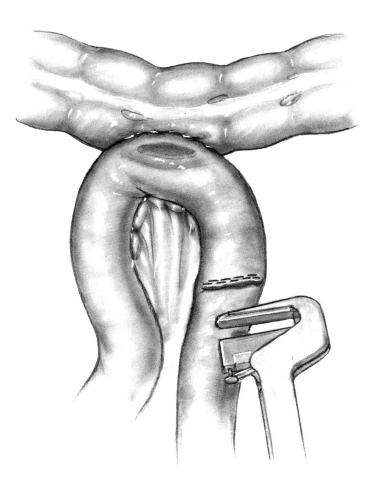

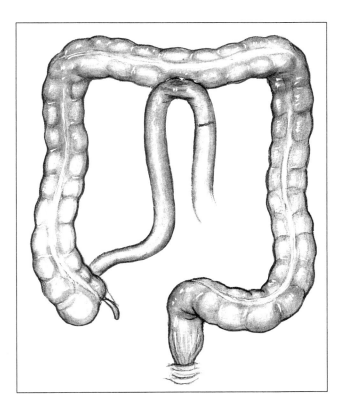

Close the EEA™ instrument and fire the staples. Inspect the anastomotic staple line for hemostasis prior to transverse closure of the ileotomy with the TA® 30 instrument.

The fascia and skin are closed in the usual manner with the DFS™ instrument and the PREMIUM® skin stapler.

Right Hemicolectomy

Auto Suture® Instruments Used in a
Right Hemicolectomy

See Cautions and Contraindications on page 236

INSTRUMENT	CLINICAL APPLICATION
LDS™ Instrument	Ligation and division of the mesenteric vessels.
EEA™ Instrument or PREMIUM CEEA™ Instrument	Anastomosis of the ileum to the colon.
TA® 55 Instrument	Closure of the colon. Alternate technique: Closure of the common opening.
GIA™ Instrument	Alternate technique: Closure and transection of the ileum and transverse colon. Anastomosis of the ileum to the colon.
DFS™ Instrument and PREMIUM® Skin Stapler	Closure of fascia and skin.

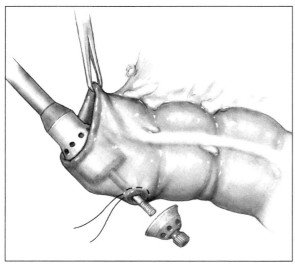

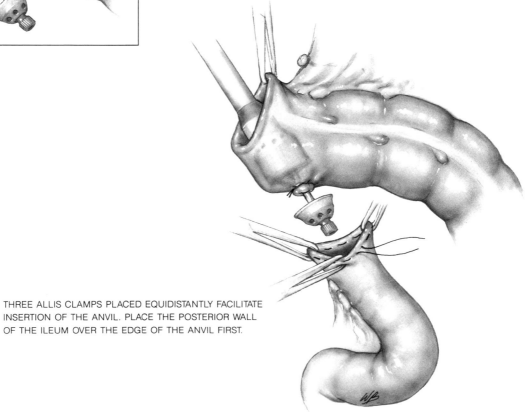

THREE ALLIS CLAMPS PLACED EQUIDISTANTLY FACILITATE
INSERTION OF THE ANVIL. PLACE THE POSTERIOR WALL
OF THE ILEUM OVER THE EDGE OF THE ANVIL FIRST.

The right colon is mobilized using the LDS™ instrument
and resected in the usual manner. The terminal ileum is
prepared with a purse string suture and the diameter of
the lumen determined using the S-EEA™ sizers.

The EEA™ instrument is used to perform the ileocolostomy.

Introduce the instrument, without anvil, into the lumen of
the transverse colon through the open transected end.
Advance the center rod through an antimesenteric stab
wound surrounded by a purse string suture. Tie the suture
and place the anvil on the center rod. Introduce the anvil
into the lumen of the ileum.

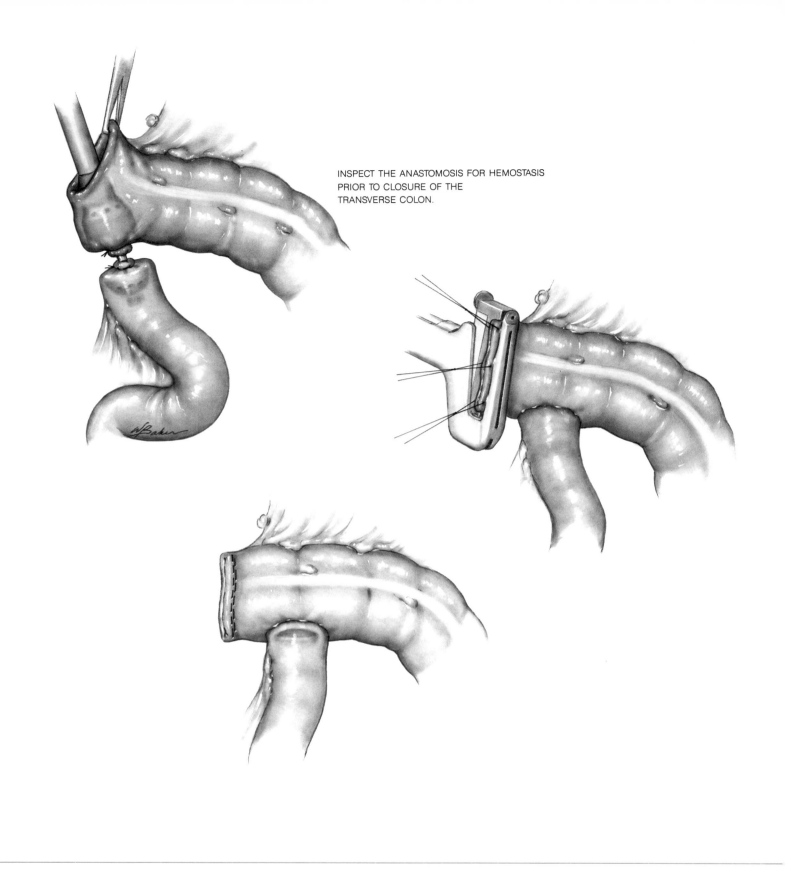

INSPECT THE ANASTOMOSIS FOR HEMOSTASIS PRIOR TO CLOSURE OF THE TRANSVERSE COLON.

Tie the purse string suture, close the EEA™ instrument and fire the staples. Open the instrument slightly and place a traction or figure-of-eight suture around the staple line. Lift the edge of the staple line over the anvil; simultaneously, gently rotate and remove the instrument. Inspect the anastomotic staple line for hemostasis prior to closure of the transverse colon with the TA® 55 instrument.

Alternate Technique

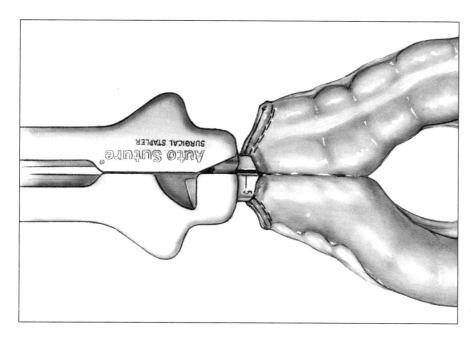

ALWAYS INSPECT THE ANASTOMOSIS
FOR HEMOSTASIS.

CARE MUST BE TAKEN TO
OVERLAP THE ENDS OF THE
PREVIOUS STAPLE LINES.

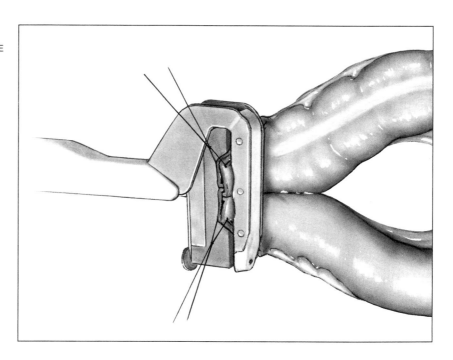

The right colon is mobilized using the LDS™
instrument and resected between two applications
of the GIA™ instrument.

The GIA™ instrument is used to perform the
ileocolostomy. Excise the antimesenteric corners of the
staple line closure of the ileum and transverse colon.

Insert one fork of the GIA™ instrument into each bowel
lumen. Close the instrument and fire the staples.
Inspect the anastomosis for hemostasis prior to closure
of the now common opening with the TA® 55 instrument.

The fascia and skin are closed in the usual manner with
the DFS™ instrument and the PREMIUM® skin stapler.

Colocolostomy

Auto Suture® Instruments Used in a Colocolostomy

See Cautions and Contraindications on page 236

INSTRUMENT	CLINICAL APPLICATION
LDS™ Instrument	Ligation and division of the mesenteric vessels.
EEA™ Instrument or PREMIUM CEEA™ Instrument	Anastomosis of the proximal and distal colon.
TA® 55 Instrument	Closure of the colotomy.
GIA™ Instrument	Alternate technique: Closure and transection of the colon.
DFS™ Instrument and PREMIUM® Skin Stapler	Closure of fascia and skin.

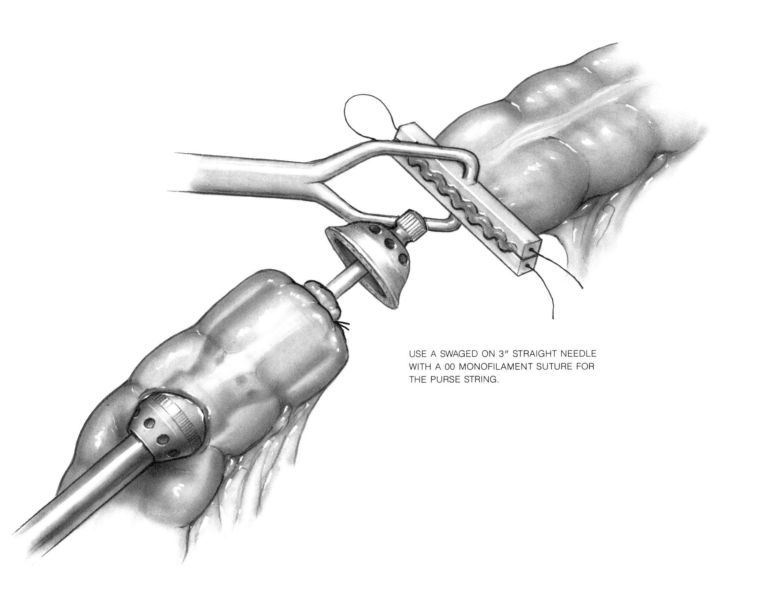

USE A SWAGED ON 3" STRAIGHT NEEDLE
WITH A 00 MONOFILAMENT SUTURE FOR
THE PURSE STRING.

The colon to be resected is mobilized using the LDS™
instrument. To prevent incorporation of staples in the
anastomosis, the LDS™ instrument may be used to
within 2 cm. of the proximal and distal points of
transection.

The purse string instrument is placed around the
proximal colon at the point of transection. The purse
string suture is applied and the colon is transected
using the instrument as a cutting guide. The diameter
of the colon is determined using the S-EEA™ sizers.

The EEA™ instrument is introduced through a colotomy
performed 3-4 cm. proximal to the anastomotic site.
Open the EEA™ instrument to advance the anvil, and
tie the purse string suture.

Place the purse string instrument around the distal
colon, apply the purse string suture and resect the
specimen.

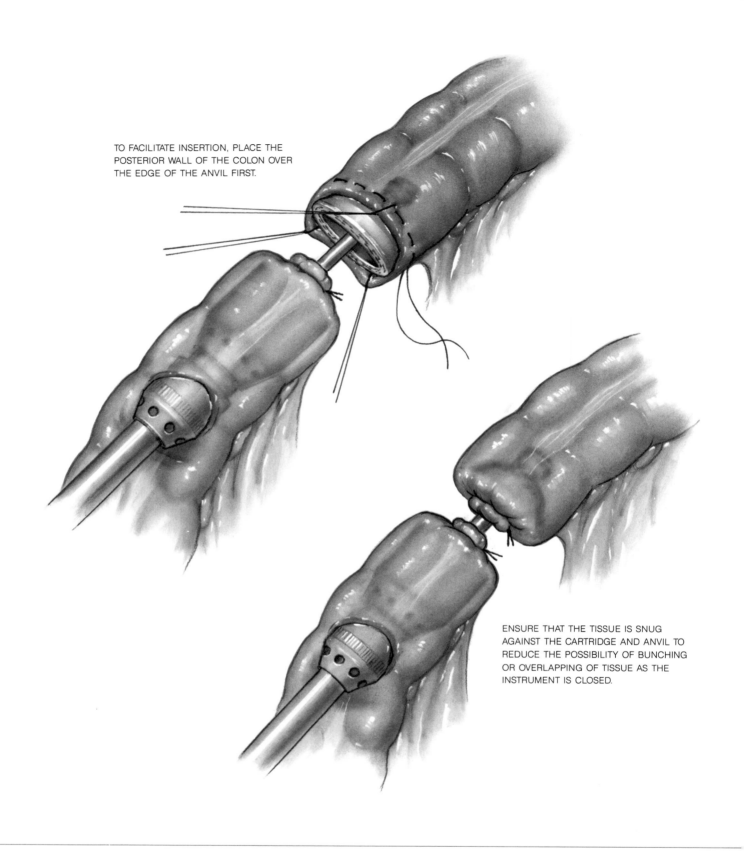

TO FACILITATE INSERTION, PLACE THE POSTERIOR WALL OF THE COLON OVER THE EDGE OF THE ANVIL FIRST.

ENSURE THAT THE TISSUE IS SNUG AGAINST THE CARTRIDGE AND ANVIL TO REDUCE THE POSSIBILITY OF BUNCHING OR OVERLAPPING OF TISSUE AS THE INSTRUMENT IS CLOSED.

Remove the purse string instrument on the distal colon and grasp the tissue edges with three traction sutures or three Allis clamps placed equidistantly just behind the purse string suture line. Introduce the anvil into the distal colon and tie the purse string suture. Close the EEA™ instrument and fire the staples.

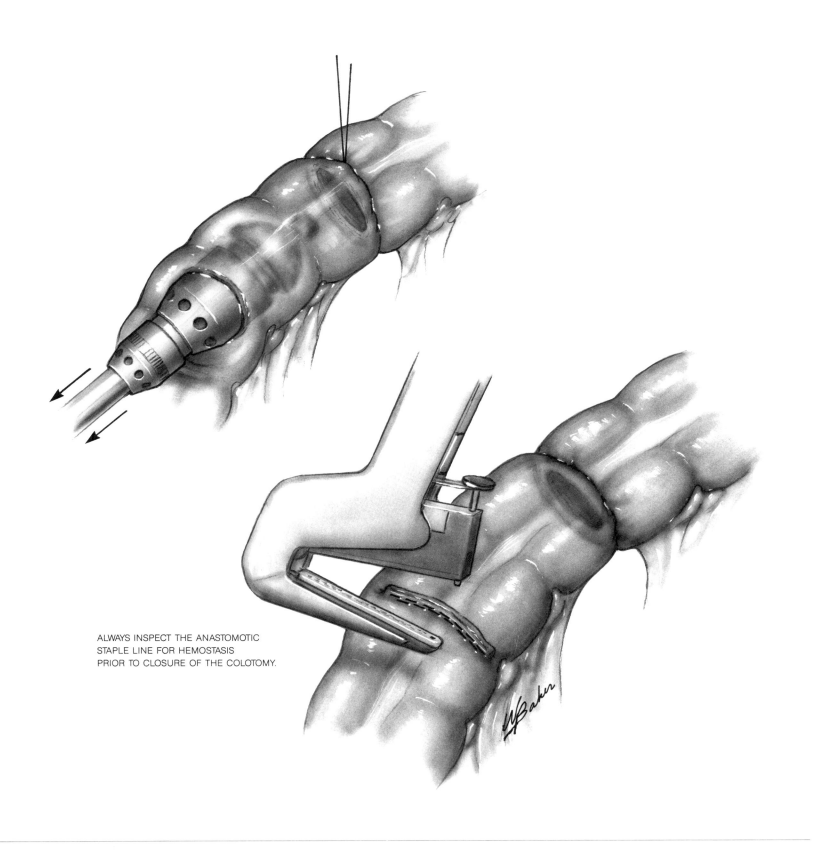

ALWAYS INSPECT THE ANASTOMOTIC
STAPLE LINE FOR HEMOSTASIS
PRIOR TO CLOSURE OF THE COLOTOMY.

Open the instrument slightly, place a traction or figure-of-eight suture around the staple line and lift the edge of the staple line over the anvil. Gently rotate and remove the instrument. Inspect the staple line for hemostasis prior to transverse closure of the colotomy with the TA® 55 instrument.

Circular Anastomosis through Linear Staple Line

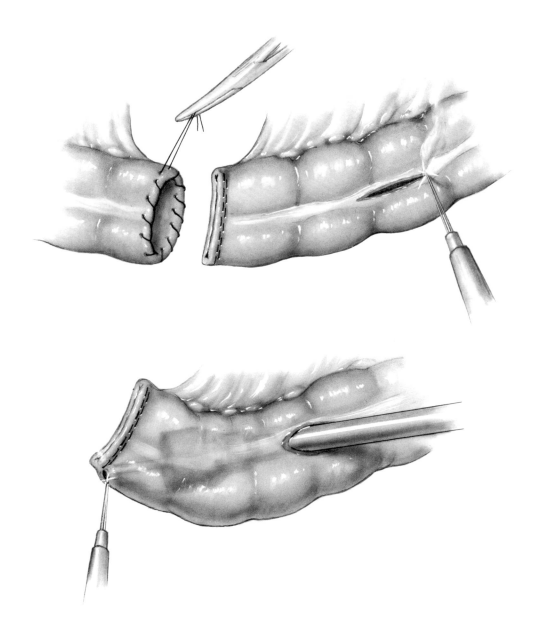

Following mobilization, the proximal colon is closed and transected using the GIA™ instrument. The distal colon is transected and prepared with a purse string suture which may be placed manually or with the purse string instrument.

The EEA™ instrument, without anvil, is introduced through a proximal colotomy. Make a small incision in or excise the antimesenteric corner of the proximal bowel at the point of transection. Place a manual purse string suture.

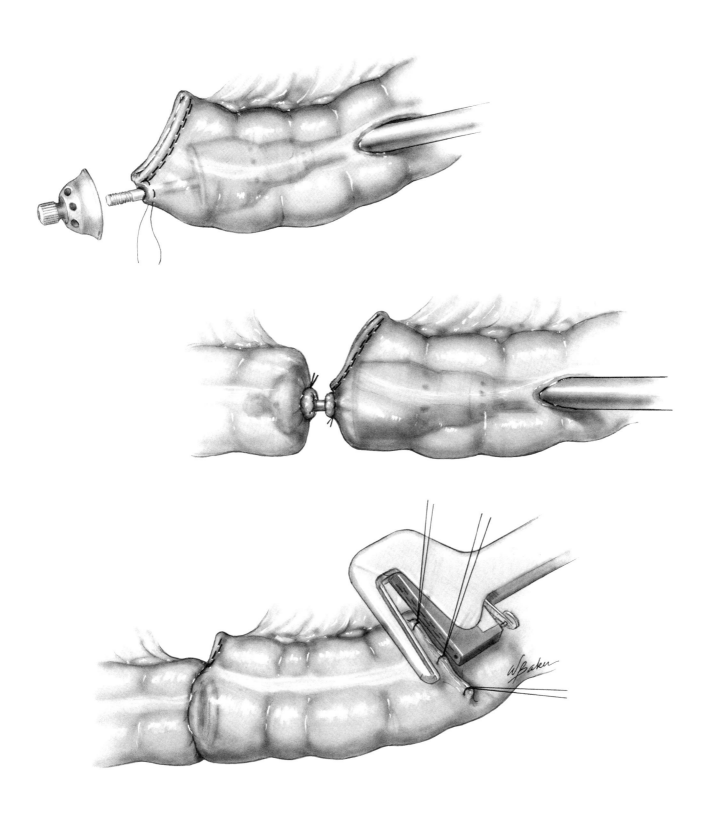

Open the EEA™ instrument to advance the center rod through the opening. Tie the purse string suture and replace the anvil.

Introduce the anvil into the distal colon and tie the purse string suture. Close the EEA™ instrument and fire the staples. Inspect the anastomotic staple line for hemostasis prior to transverse closure of the colotomy with the TA® 55 instrument.

This technique is particularly useful for anastomosis when discrepancy in bowel lumen size exists between the proximal and distal segments.

The fascia and skin are closed in the usual manner with the DFS™ instrument and the PREMIUM® skin stapler.

Colostomy

Auto Suture® Instruments Used in a Colostomy

See Cautions and Contraindications on page 236

INSTRUMENT	CLINICAL APPLICATION
PREMIUM CEEA™ Instrument or EEA™ Instrument	Creation of the colostomy.
DFS™ Instrument and PREMIUM® Skin Stapler	Closure of fascia and skin.

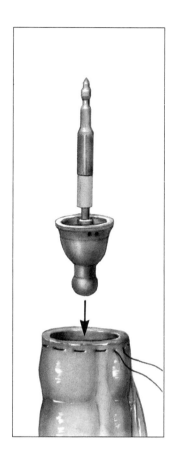

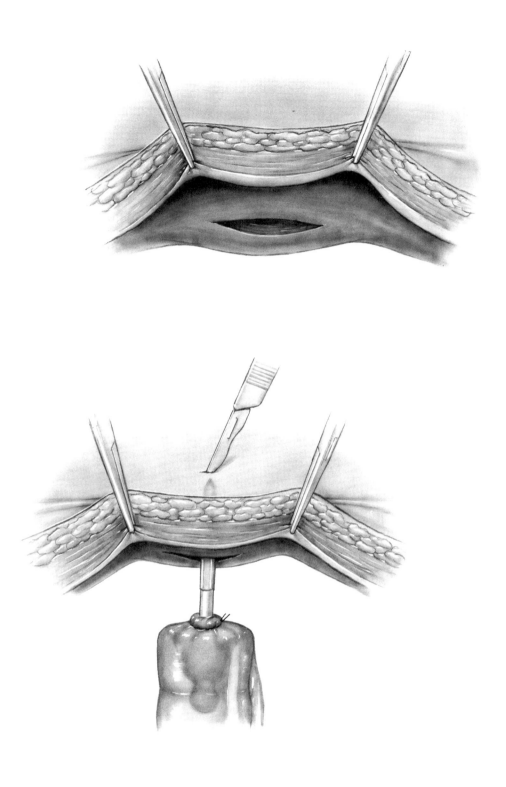

The PREMIUM CEEA™ instrument is used to create the end colostomy. The proximal colon is prepared with a purse string suture using the purse string instrument. The anvil with anvil shaft is introduced into the lumen of the proximal colon and the purse string suture is tied into the purse string notch on the anvil shaft.

The site of the colostomy is chosen and the peritoneum, muscle and fascia are incised from within over a distance sufficient to accommodate the colon. The subcutaneous tissue is spread to the level of the dermis and the anvil shaft is introduced through the incision to just beneath the skin. Incise the skin over the tip of the anvil shaft to allow passage of the shaft through the skin.

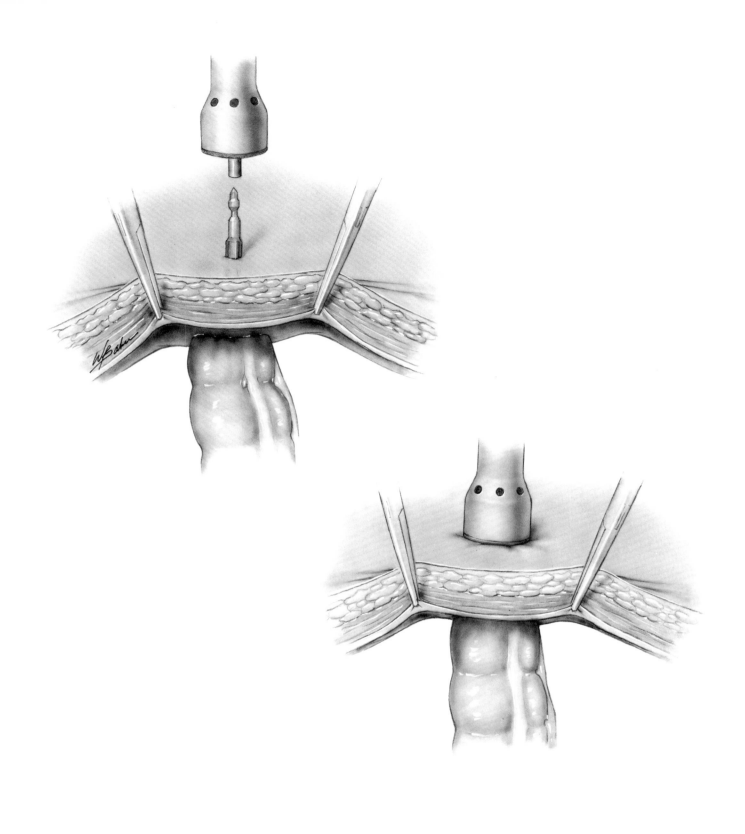

Direct the anvil and colon through the abdominal wall incision to just beneath the skin. Engage the anvil shaft in the instrument shaft. Close the instrument, fire the staples and remove the instrument.

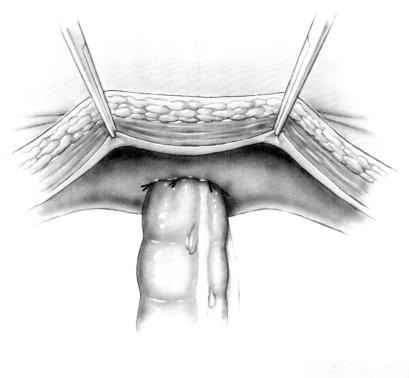

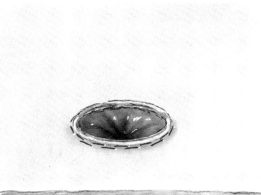

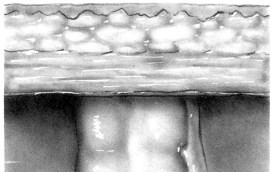

The position of the colostomy is maintained by suturing the colon to the peritoneum with interrupted sutures.

A similar technique may be used to perform an ileostomy. In this case, the ileum is everted at the skin level to create the desired stoma.

Alternate Technique

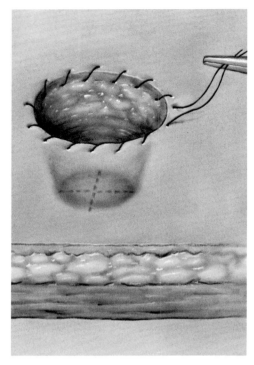

USE A 00 MONOFILAMENT
SUTURE ON A CUTTING NEEDLE
FOR THE PURSE STRING

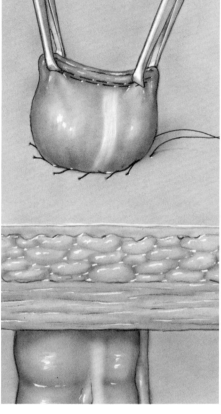

THE ABDOMINAL INCISION
MAY BE CLOSED PRIOR TO
OPENING THE BOWEL.

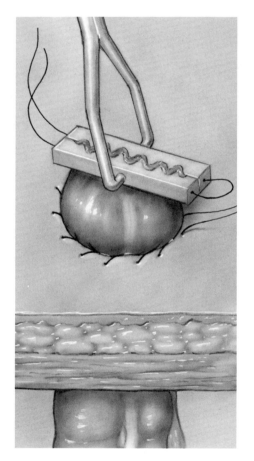

Following colon transection and preparation of the proximal bowel, a 2 cm. diameter circular incision is made into the skin at the site of the colostomy. A manual purse string suture is applied to the skin edge. The usual incision is made in the fascia and the muscle is spread or incised.

The proximal colon is presented through the incision. Place the purse string instrument and a purse string suture on the proximal colon just beneath the staple line closure. Excise the redundant tissue and staple line using the purse string instrument as a cutting guide.

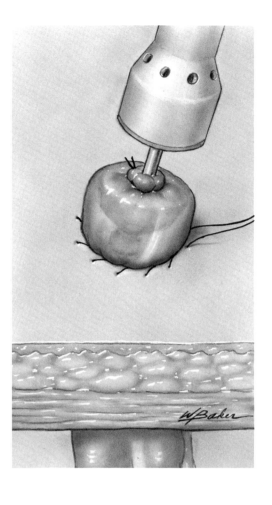

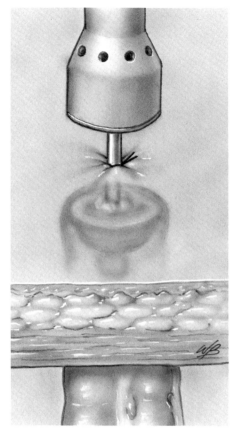

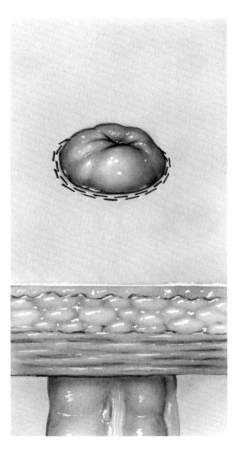

The EEA™ instrument is used to create the colostomy. Introduce the anvil into the lumen of the colon and tie the purse string suture. Place gentle downward traction on the colon to bring the anvil and colon beneath the skin edge.

Tie the purse string suture on the skin. Close the instrument, fire the staples and remove the instrument.

The fascia and skin are closed in the usual manner with the DFS™ instrument and the PREMIUM® skin stapler.

Low Anterior Resection –
End-to-End Anastomosis

Auto Suture® Instruments Used in a
Low Anterior Resection with End-to-End Anastomosis

See Cautions and Contraindications on page 236

INSTRUMENT	CLINICAL APPLICATION
LDS™ Instrument	Ligation and division of the mesenteric vessels.
GIA™ Instrument	Closure and transection of the proximal colon.
PREMIUM CEEA™ Instrument or EEA™ Instrument	Anastomosis of the proximal colon to the rectum.
ROTICULATOR® 55 Instrument	Alternate technique: Closure of the rectum.
DFS™ Instrument and PREMIUM® Skin Stapler	Closure of fascia and skin.

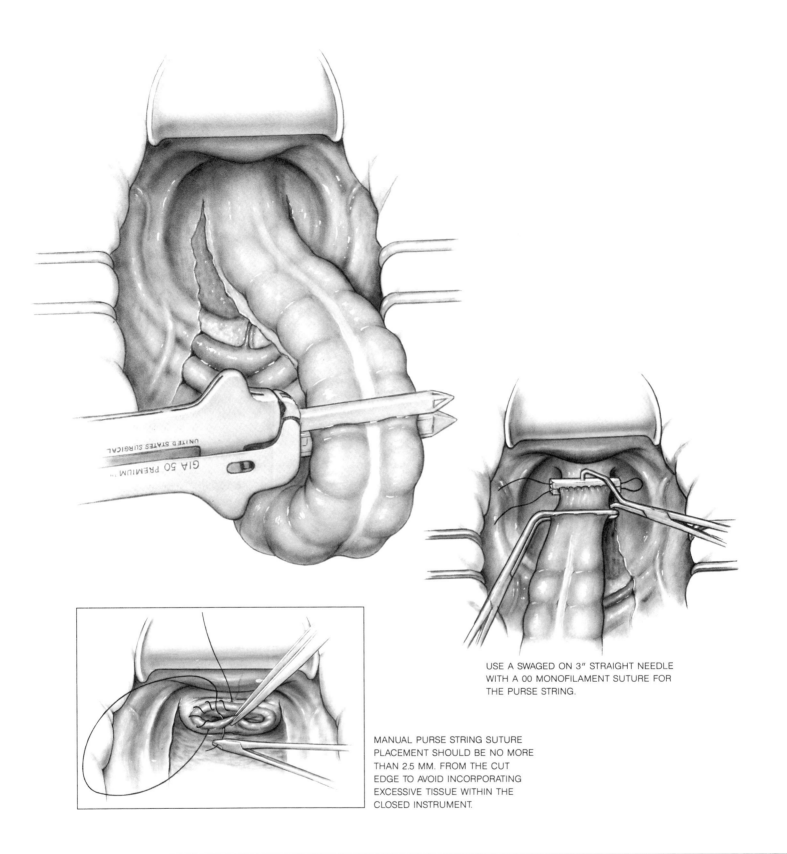

USE A SWAGED ON 3″ STRAIGHT NEEDLE
WITH A 00 MONOFILAMENT SUTURE FOR
THE PURSE STRING.

MANUAL PURSE STRING SUTURE
PLACEMENT SHOULD BE NO MORE
THAN 2.5 MM. FROM THE CUT
EDGE TO AVOID INCORPORATING
EXCESSIVE TISSUE WITHIN THE
CLOSED INSTRUMENT.

The colon to be resected is mobilized using the LDS™ instrument. To prevent incorporation of staples in the anastomosis, the LDS™ instrument may be used to within 2 cm. of the proximal and distal points of transection. The GIA™ instrument is used to close and transect the proximal colon.

The purse string instrument is applied around the rectum utilizing the specimen for traction as necessary. Place the purse string suture and resect the specimen using the purse string instrument edge as a cutting guide.

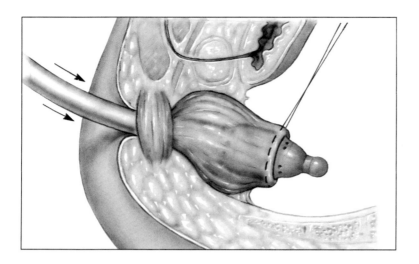

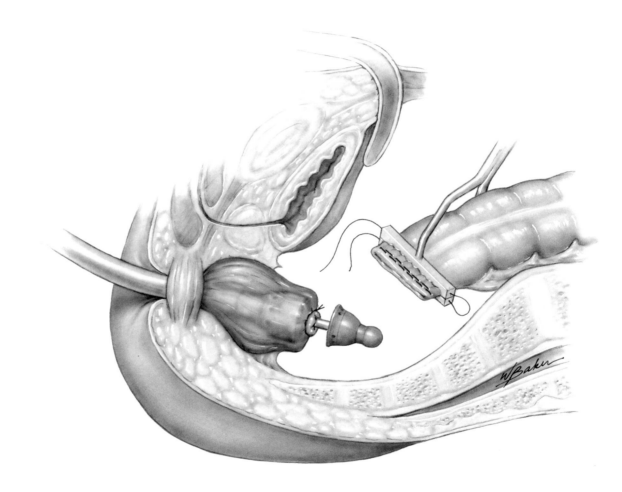

The PREMIUM CEEA™ instrument is used to perform the anastomosis. Introduce the instrument transanally and advance the instrument to the level of the purse string instrument. Remove the purse string instrument, open the PREMIUM CEEA™ instrument allowing the anvil to protrude from the rectum and tie the rectal purse string suture.

Apply the purse string instrument around the proximal colon just above the staple line closure. Place the purse string suture and resect the excess tissue using the instrument edge as a cutting guide.

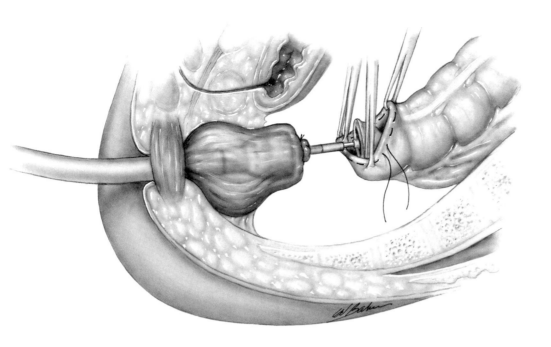

Alternate Technique

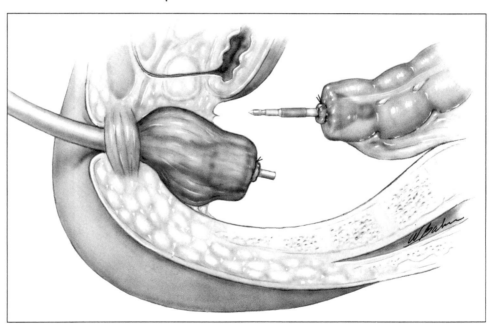

Remove the purse string instrument and grasp the tissue edges with three Allis clamps placed equidistantly. Introduce the anvil of the instrument into the proximal colon and tie the purse string suture.

In an alternate technique, the proximal colon may be prepared with the anvil and anvil shaft separated from the instrument. The instrument, without anvil, is introduced transanally to the level of the purse string suture. The instrument is opened and the purse string suture is tied. The anvil shaft is then engaged in the instrument shaft.

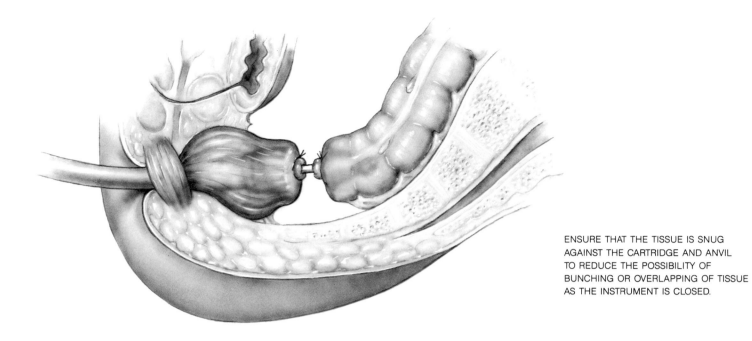

ENSURE THAT THE TISSUE IS SNUG
AGAINST THE CARTRIDGE AND ANVIL
TO REDUCE THE POSSIBILITY OF
BUNCHING OR OVERLAPPING OF TISSUE
AS THE INSTRUMENT IS CLOSED.

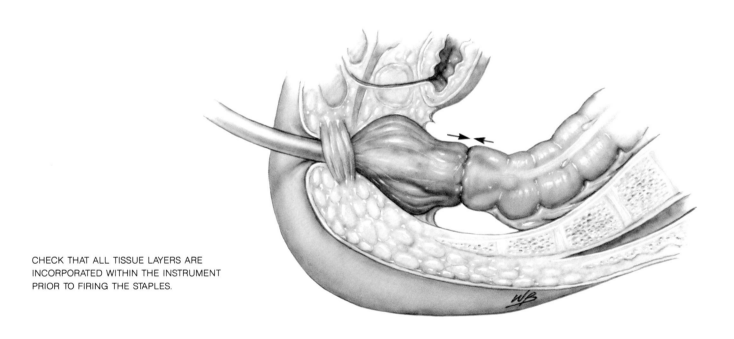

CHECK THAT ALL TISSUE LAYERS ARE
INCORPORATED WITHIN THE INSTRUMENT
PRIOR TO FIRING THE STAPLES.

Close the PREMIUM CEEA™ instrument and fire the staples. A circular double staggered row of staples joins the bowel and the circular blade in the instrument cuts a stoma.

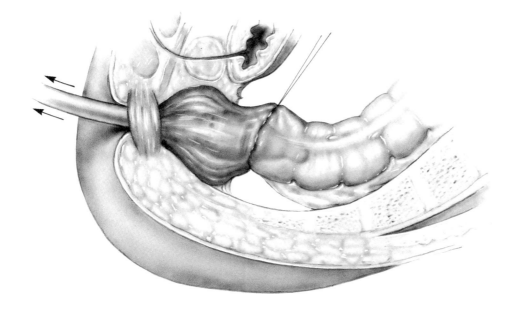

INSPECT THE TISSUE
WITHIN THE CARTRIDGE FOR
CONTINUITY OF THE PURSE
STRING SUTURES AND PRESENCE
OF ALL TISSUE LAYERS

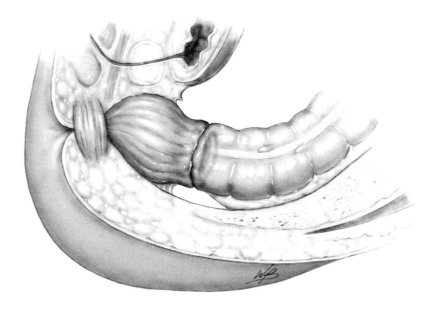

USING A SCOPE, INSPECT THE
ANASTOMOTIC STAPLE LINE FOR
HEMOSTASIS.

Open the instrument slightly and place a traction or figure-of-eight suture around the staple line. Lift the staple line over the anvil; simultaneously, gently rotate and remove the instrument.

The resulting anastomosis is illustrated with the bowel wall transparent to depict the reconstruction.

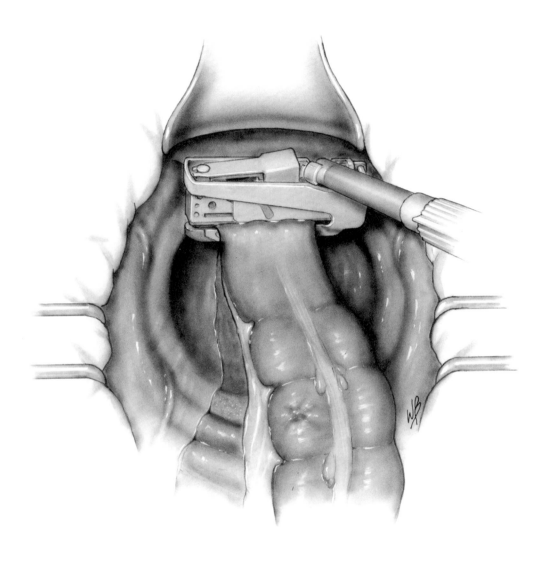

The segment of colon to be resected is mobilized using the LDS™ instrument to ligate and divide the mesocolon.

The rectum is closed with the ROTICULATOR® 55 instrument. Slip the jaws of the instrument around the rectum at the point of transection. Close the instrument and fire the staples. Prior to removing the instrument, place a clamp on the specimen side and transect the rectum using the ROTICULATOR® 55 instrument edge as a cutting guide.

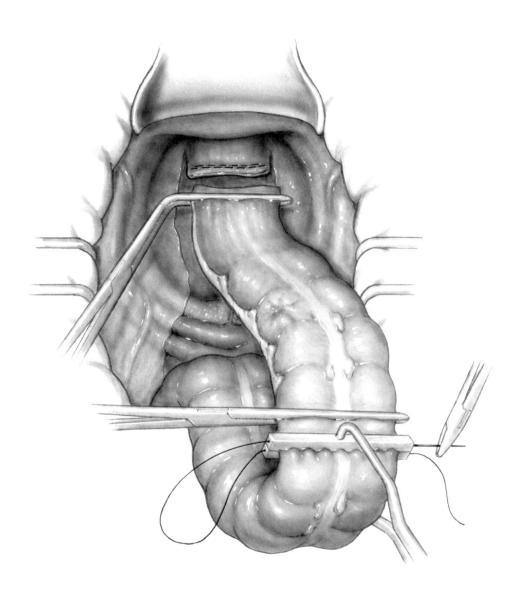

The purse string instrument is used to place a purse string suture on the proximal colon. Place a clamp on the specimen side and transect the colon using the purse string instrument as a cutting guide.

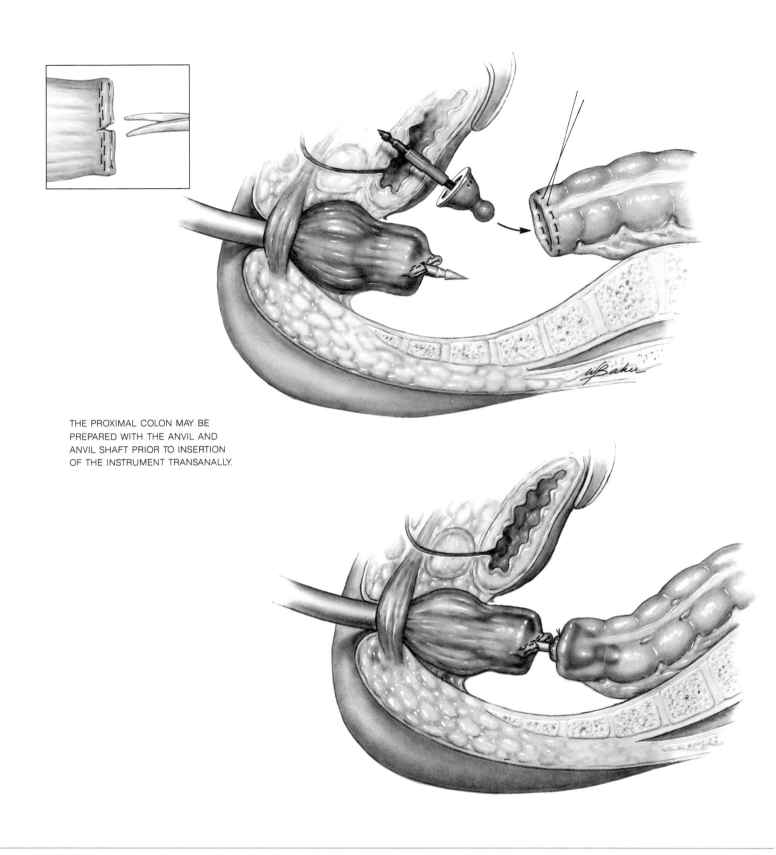

THE PROXIMAL COLON MAY BE
PREPARED WITH THE ANVIL AND
ANVIL SHAFT PRIOR TO INSERTION
OF THE INSTRUMENT TRANSANALLY.

The PREMIUM CEEA™ instrument is used to perform the colorectal anastomosis. Introduce the instrument, without anvil and anvil shaft and with recessed trocar tip, transanally. Advance the instrument to the staple line closure of the rectum. Using scissors, make a small incision into the rectum through the staple line at the midpoint of the closure. Fully advance the trocar tip through the incision and remove the trocar tip using a Babcock clamp.

Remove the purse string instrument, introduce the anvil with the anvil shaft into the lumen of the proximal colon and tie the purse string suture. Engage the anvil shaft in the instrument shaft.

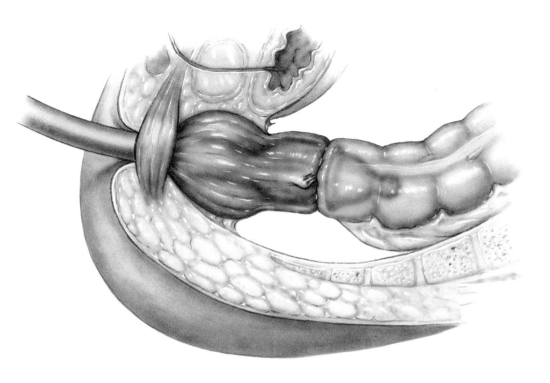

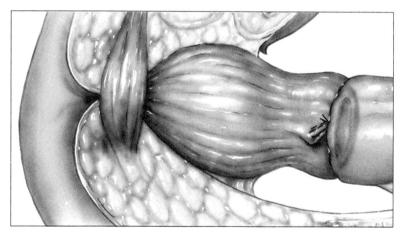

ALWAYS INSPECT THE ANASTOMOTIC
STAPLE LINE FOR HEMOSTASIS.

Close the PREMIUM CEEA™ instrument and fire the staples. Open the instrument slightly and place a traction or figure-of-eight suture around the staple line. Lift the edge of the staple line over the anvil; simultaneously, gently rotate and remove the instrument. Using a scope, inspect the anastomotic staple line for hemostasis.

The fascia and skin are closed in the usual manner with the DFS™ instrument and PREMIUM® skin stapler.

Low Anterior Resection –
Side-to-Side Anastomosis

Auto Suture® Instruments Used in a
Low Anterior Resection with Side-to-Side Anastomosis

See Cautions and Contraindications on page 236

INSTRUMENT	CLINICAL APPLICATION
LDS™ Instrument	Ligation and division of the mesenteric vessels.
GIA™ Instrument	Closure and transection of the proximal colon. Anastomosis of the proximal colon to the rectum.
TA® 55 Instrument	Alternate closure of the proximal colon.
ROTICULATOR® 55 Instrument	Closure of the rectum and colonic stab wound.
DFS™ Instrument and PREMIUM® Skin Stapler	Closure of fascia and skin.

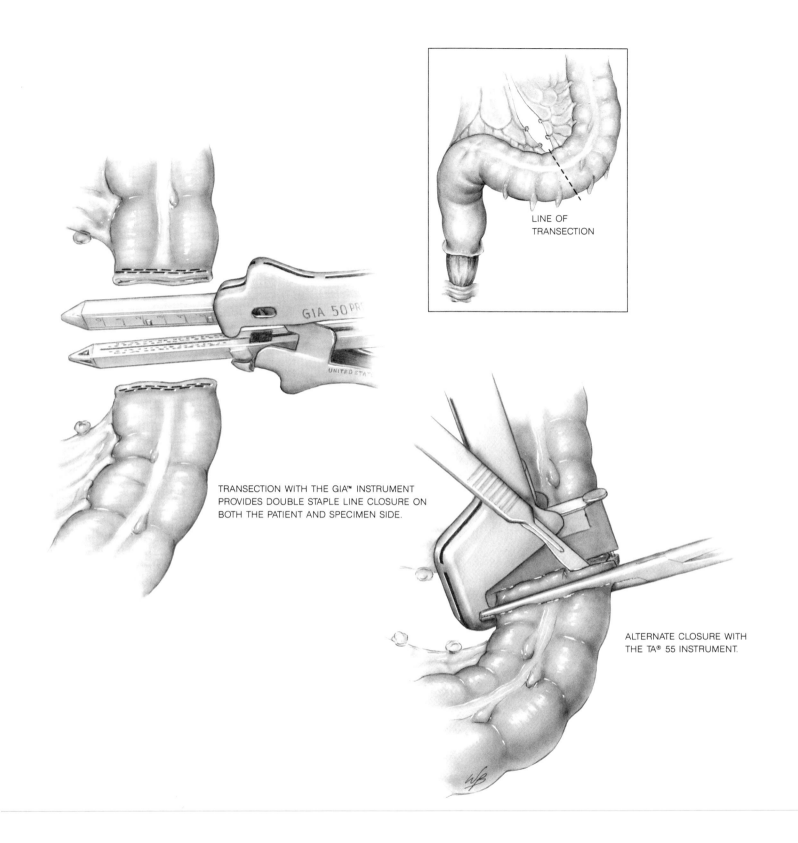

LINE OF
TRANSECTION

TRANSECTION WITH THE GIA™ INSTRUMENT
PROVIDES DOUBLE STAPLE LINE CLOSURE ON
BOTH THE PATIENT AND SPECIMEN SIDE.

ALTERNATE CLOSURE WITH
THE TA® 55 INSTRUMENT.

The segment of colon to be resected is mobilized using the LDS™ instrument to ligate and divide the mesenteric vessels. The LDS™ instrument may be employed to ligate and divide the vascular perirectal fatty tissue during mobilization of the rectum.

The proximal colon is closed with either the GIA™ instrument or the TA® 55 instrument. Position the bowel so that the mesocolon will be on the posterior wall of the proximal colon opposite the anastomotic site.

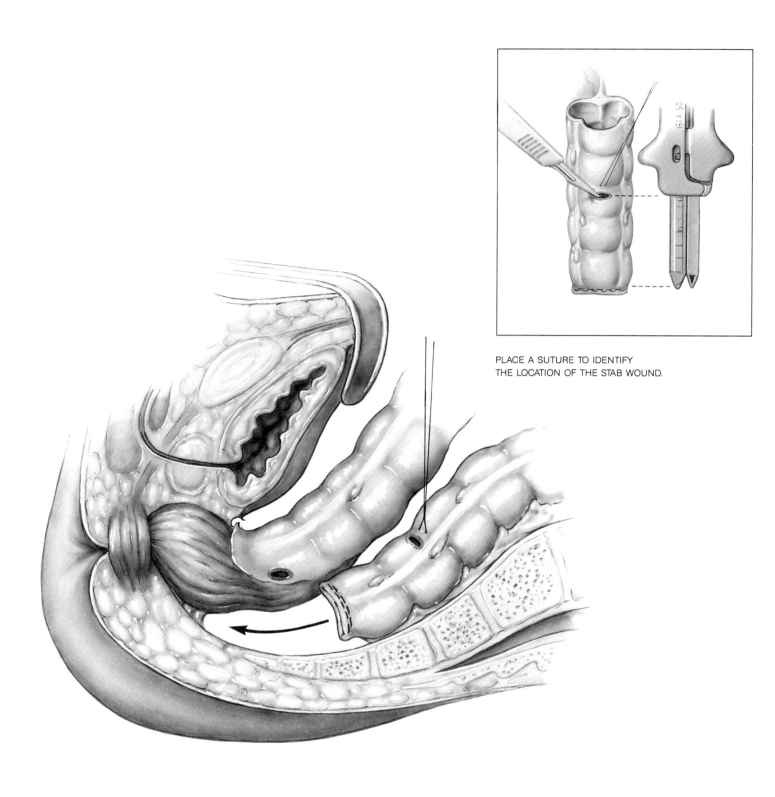

PLACE A SUTURE TO IDENTIFY
THE LOCATION OF THE STAB WOUND.

Dissection is carried down behind the rectum.

The GIA™ instrument is used to perform the colorectal anastomosis. Make a 1 cm. stab wound into the anti-mesenteric border of the colon 5 cm. proximal to the staple line closure. Use the fork of the GIA™ instrument as a measuring device to facilitate stab wound placement.

Make a corresponding stab wound into the left anterolateral wall of the rectum at the proximal point of the planned site of anastomosis.

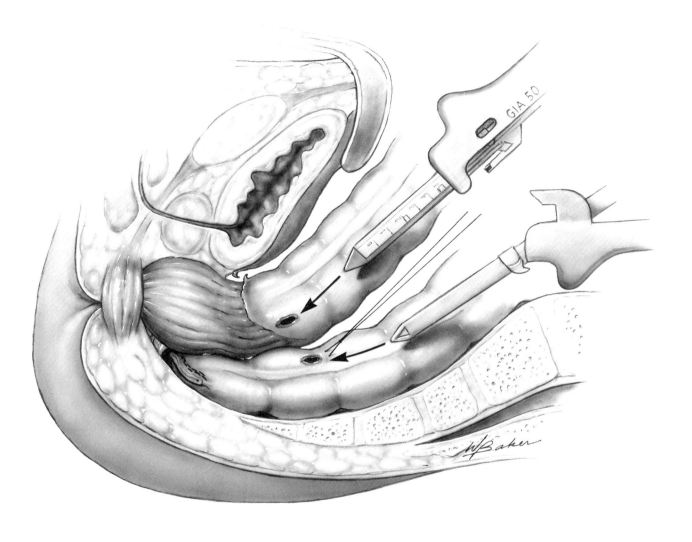

The proximal colon is placed into the retrorectal space. Gentle traction on the specimen elevates the rectum and facilitates placement of the GIA™ instrument.

Insert the cartridge fork of the GIA™ instrument into the rectum and the anvil fork into the lumen of the colon.

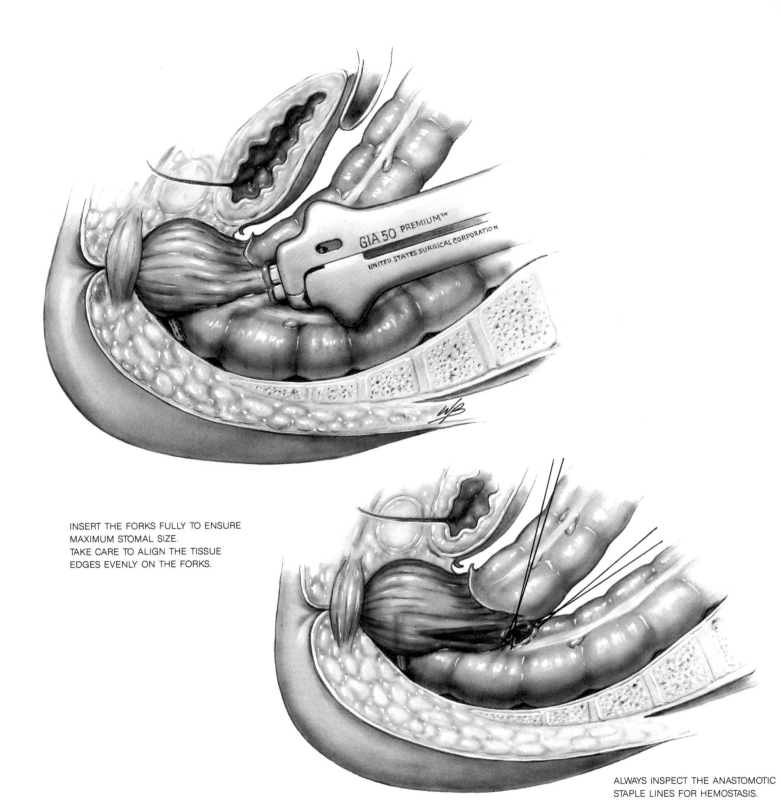

INSERT THE FORKS FULLY TO ENSURE
MAXIMUM STOMAL SIZE.
TAKE CARE TO ALIGN THE TISSUE
EDGES EVENLY ON THE FORKS.

ALWAYS INSPECT THE ANASTOMOTIC
STAPLE LINES FOR HEMOSTASIS.

Close the instrument and fire the staples. Two double staggered staple lines join the posterior rectal wall to the anterior colonic wall; simultaneously, the knife blade cuts between the staple lines, dividing the spur and creating a common colorectal cavity.

Inspect the anastomotic staple lines for hemostasis prior to closure of the common stab wound and rectum and resection of the specimen. Place an everting traction suture around each anastomotic staple line and hold the staple lines apart.

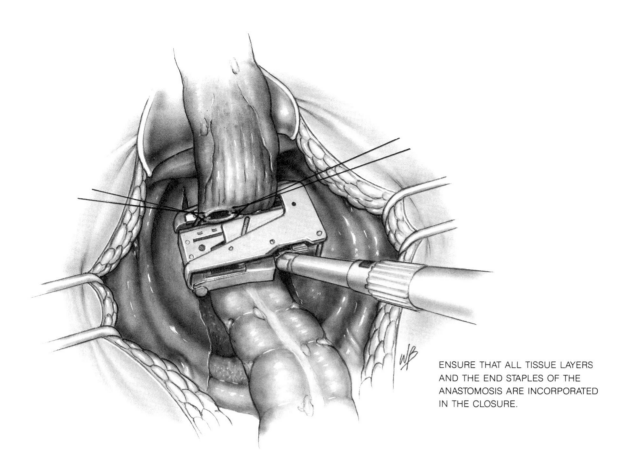

ENSURE THAT ALL TISSUE LAYERS
AND THE END STAPLES OF THE
ANASTOMOSIS ARE INCORPORATED
IN THE CLOSURE.

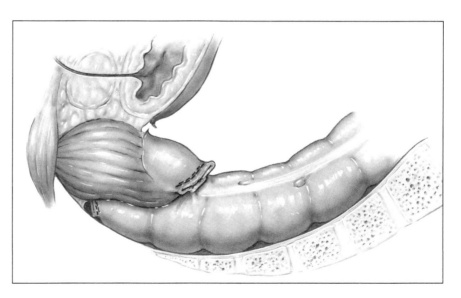

To simultaneously close the now common stab wound and rectum, place the ROTICULATOR® 55 instrument around the rectum and beneath the two traction sutures. Care is taken to include the two lips of the common stab wound on the specimen side of the instrument. Close the instrument and fire the staples.

Resect the specimen using the instrument edge as a cutting guide prior to removing the instrument.

The fascia and skin are closed in the usual manner with the DFS™ instrument and the PREMIUM® skin stapler.

Duhamel Procedure

Auto Suture® Instruments Used in a Duhamel Procedure

See Cautions and Contraindications on page 236

INSTRUMENT	CLINICAL APPLICATION
LDS™ Instrument	Ligation and division of the mesenteric vessels.
GIA™ Instrument	Closure and transection of the proximal colon. Anastomosis of the colon to the rectum.
TA® 30 Instrument or TA® 55 Instrument	Closure of the rectum. Closure of the colotomy.
PREMIUM CEEA™ Instrument or EEA™ Instrument	Anastomosis of the colon to the rectum.
PREMIUM® Skin Stapler	Closure of skin.

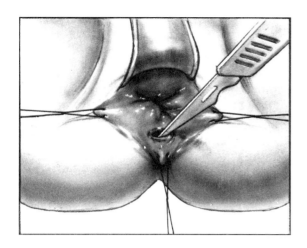

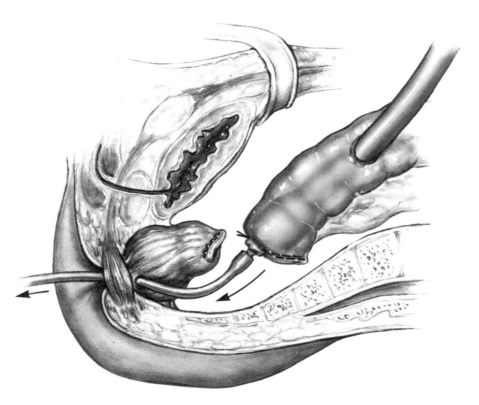

The segment of colon to be resected is mobilized using the LDS™ instrument to ligate and divide the corresponding mesocolon. The proximal colon is closed and transected using the GIA™ instrument. The rectum is closed with the TA® 30 instrument or TA® 55 instrument and the aganglionic bowel is resected. A retro-rectal tunnel is created and a stab wound is made into the posterior anal wall approximately 1-1.5 cm. above the pectinate line. A #14 or #16 red rubber catheter is placed from above, downward into the retrorectal tunnel and out through the stab wound.

The PREMIUM CEEA™ instrument, without anvil, is introduced through a proximal colotomy approximately 8 cm. from the staple line closure of the colon. Excise the antimesocolic corner of the staple line and place a purse string suture. Advance the anvil shaft through the opening and tie the suture. Attach the flange of the catheter to the anvil shaft of the instrument. Bring the proximal colon down into the retrorectal space and guide the anvil shaft through the anal stab wound.

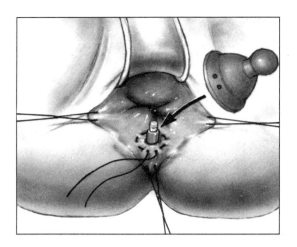

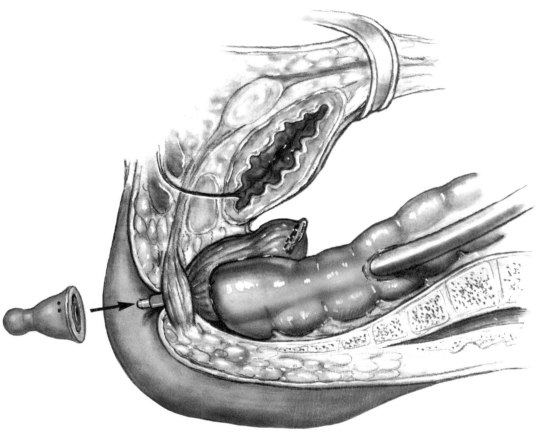

Place a purse string suture in the anal tissue around the anvil shaft. Tie the suture and place the anvil on the instrument.

Close the instrument and fire the staples. Inspect the anastomotic staple line for hemostasis.

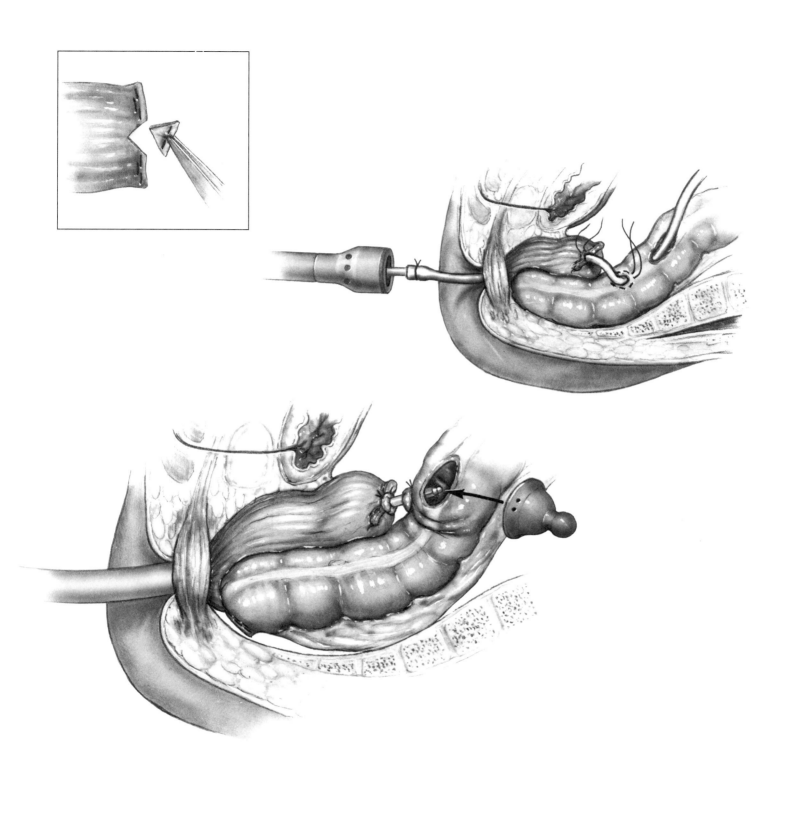

Excise the center of the rectal stump closure and apply a purse string suture. Incise the anterior wall of the proximal colon at the level of the rectal stump and place a second purse string suture. Pass a guiding catheter from the anus, through the rectal stump opening, into the distal colon incision and out the more proximal colotomy. Attach the flange of the catheter to the anvil shaft of the instrument. Introduce

the PREMIUM CEEA™ instrument, without anvil, into the rectum and guide the anvil shaft through the rectal stump opening. Advance the anvil shaft and tie the purse string suture.

Guide the anvil shaft into the colon and tie the purse string suture. Through the proximal colotomy, remove the catheter and place the anvil on the anvil shaft.

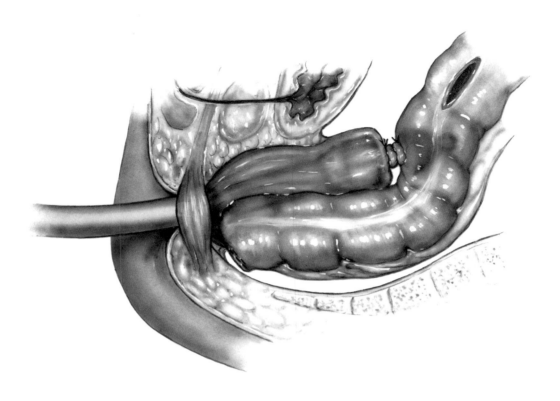

Close the instrument and fire the staples. Inspect the
anastomotic staple line for hemostasis.

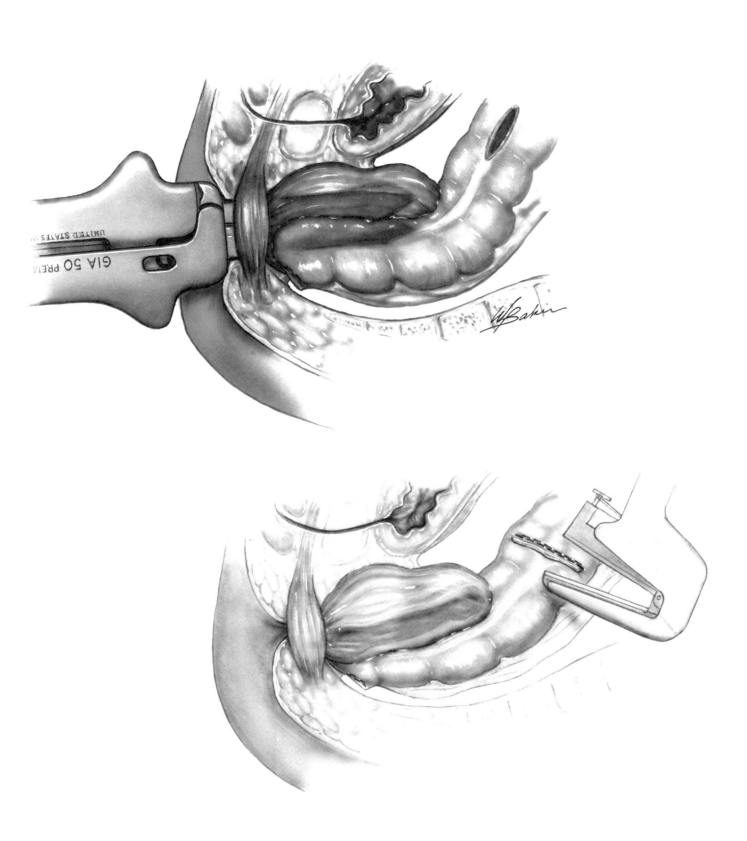

The GIA™ instrument is used to complete the colorectal anastomosis between the two circular openings. Insert one fork of the instrument into the rectum and one fork into the retrorectal colon. Close the instrument and fire the staples. Inspect the anastomotic staple lines for hemostasis prior to transverse closure of the colotomy with the TA® 30 instrument or TA® 55 instrument.

The skin is closed in the usual manner with the PREMIUM® skin stapler.

Ileal "J" Pouch

Auto Suture® Instruments Used in an Ileal "J" Pouch

See Cautions and Contraindications on page 236

INSTRUMENT	CLINICAL APPLICATION
LDS™ Instrument	Ligation and division of the mesenteric vessels.
GIA™ Instrument	Closure and transection of the terminal ileum. Anastomosis of the ileal loop forming the pouch.
EEA™ Instrument or PREMIUM CEEA™ Instrument	Anastomosis of the ileal pouch to the anal canal.
DFS™ Instrument and PREMIUM® Skin Stapler	Closure of fascia and skin.

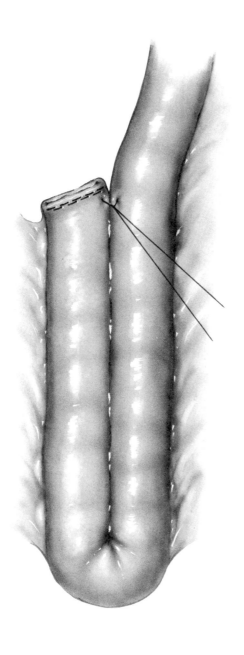

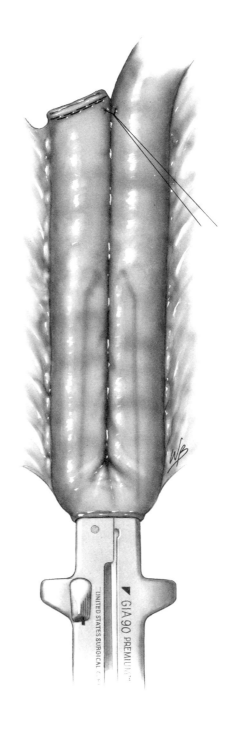

The colon is mobilized using the LDS™ instrument and a total colectomy is performed leaving a 5-6 cm. rectal pouch. The terminal ileum is closed and transected using the GIA™ instrument. The mesentery is further mobilized to allow the ileal reservoir to reach the anus without tension.

The distal 25-40 cm. of ileum is looped approximating the antimesenteric borders of the bowel, forming a "J" loop with 12-20 cm. limbs.

The GIA™ instrument is used to create the ileal pouch. Make a stab wound into the antimesenteric border of the ileum at the apex of the loop. Insert one fork of the instrument into each bowel limb. Close the instrument and fire the staples. Repeat the procedure using the same opening until the pouch construction is complete. Care must be taken to incorporate the end staples of the previous application to ensure continuity of the staple lines. Inspect the anastomotic staple lines for hemostasis.

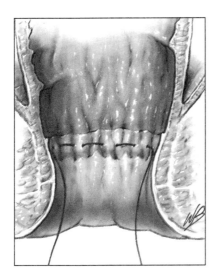

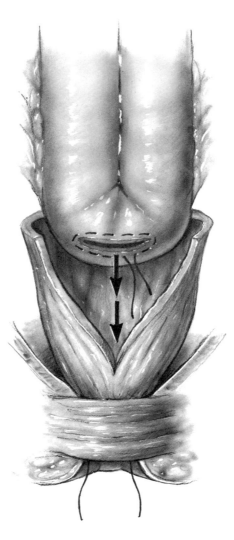

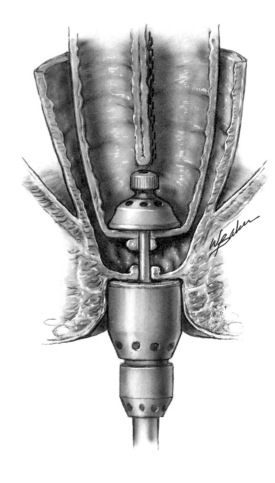

The distal rectal mucosectomy is performed.

The EEA™ instrument may be used to perform the ileoanal anastomosis. A manual purse string suture is placed around the ileal stab wound and a second manual purse string suture is placed 0.5 cm. above the dentate line. The rectum is incised longitudinally to accommodate the ileal pouch.

Introduce the EEA™ instrument into the anus and advance the center rod. Tie the anal purse string suture. Insert the anvil into the lumen of the pouch and tie the ileal purse string suture. Close the instrument and fire the staples. Inspect the anastomosis for hemostasis.

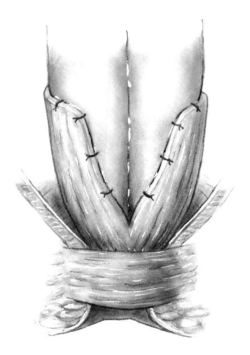

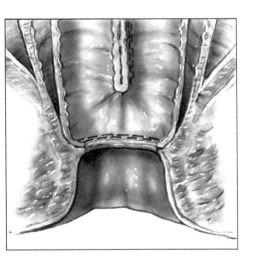

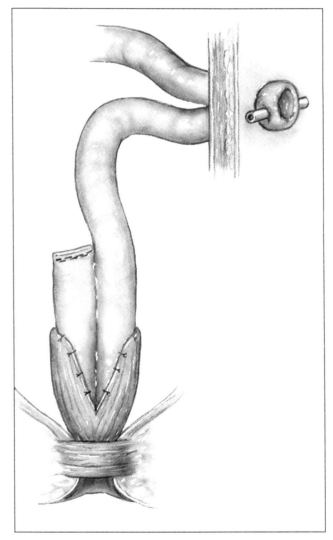

The ileal pouch is secured to the rectal muscularis with interrupted sutures.

A proximal diverting loop ileostomy is performed and maintained until complete healing of the neorectum and anastomosis is demonstrated.

The fascia and skin are closed in the usual manner with the DFS™ instrument and the PREMIUM® skin stapler.

Kock Ileal Reservoir

Auto Suture® Instruments Used in a Kock Ileal Reservoir

See Cautions and Contraindications on page 236

INSTRUMENT	CLINICAL APPLICATION
GIA™ Instrument	Closure and transection of the terminal ileum. Creation of the posterior wall of the pouch. Secure shape of the nipple.
TA® 90 Instrument	Closure of the lateral walls of the pouch.
DFS™ Instrument and PREMIUM® Skin Stapler	Closure of fascia and skin.

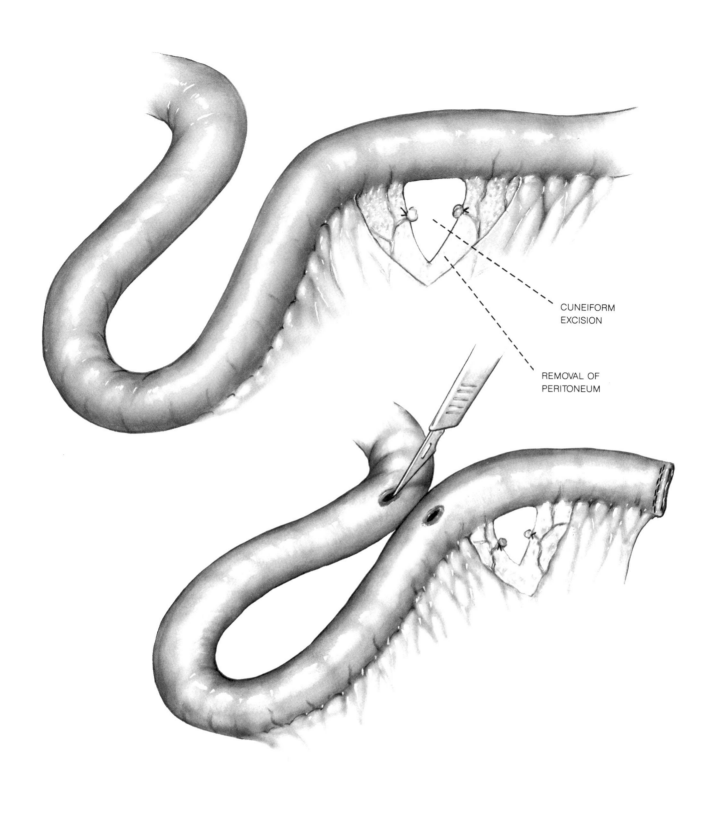

CUNEIFORM
EXCISION

REMOVAL OF
PERITONEUM

The terminal ileum is closed and transected using the GIA™ instrument.

The mesentery of the terminal ileum is transilluminated to outline the vessels and determine the segment to be used for the nipple valve construction. An opening is made in an avascular area of the mesentery 5-10 cm. from the terminal end. The visceral peritoneum on both sides of the mesentery and a portion of the

mesenteric fat are removed to reduce the bulk of mesentery to be intussuscepted.

To construct the ileal reservoir, a bowel segment of 30 cm. is folded in a U-shaped fashion leaving a distal segment of 10 cm. for the nipple and stoma. Parallel stab wounds are made in the antimesenteric borders of the apposed bowel segments 15 cm. from the distal end of the loop.

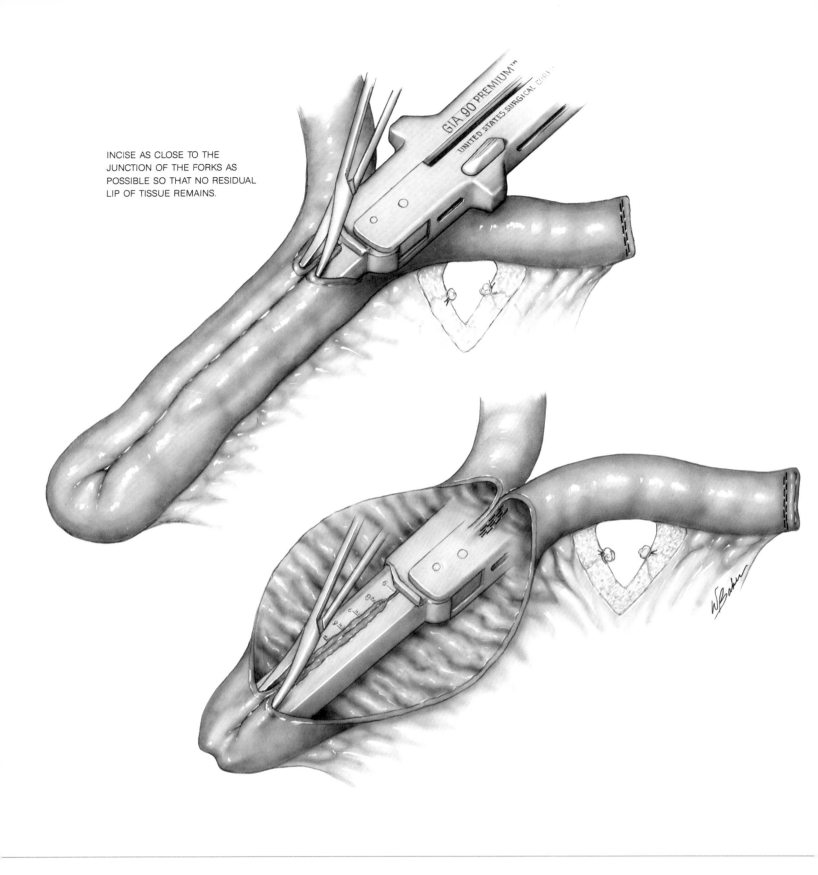

INCISE AS CLOSE TO THE
JUNCTION OF THE FORKS AS
POSSIBLE SO THAT NO RESIDUAL
LIP OF TISSUE REMAINS.

The GIA™ instrument is utilized with the SGIA™ loading unit which contains <u>no knife</u> in the push-bar assembly, placing four parallel rows of staples without dividing the tissue. Insert one fork of the instrument into each bowel lumen, close the instrument and fire the staples. Prior to removing the instrument, use the forks as a cutting guide to incise the anterior bowel walls for the length of the staple line. Reapply the instrument to complete the posterior wall of the pouch. Care must be taken to incorporate the end staples of the previous application to ensure continuity of the staple lines. With the final application, place the forks well beyond the septum to ensure complete tissue closure.

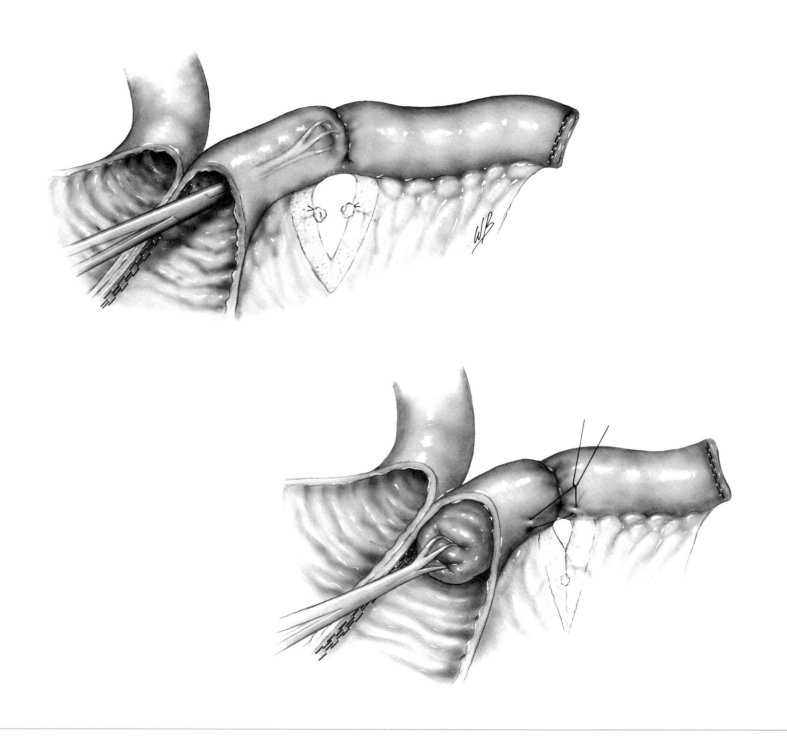

In preparation for the nipple construction, care must be taken to intussuscept the bowel wall sufficiently to position the nipple well within the lumen of the future reservoir.

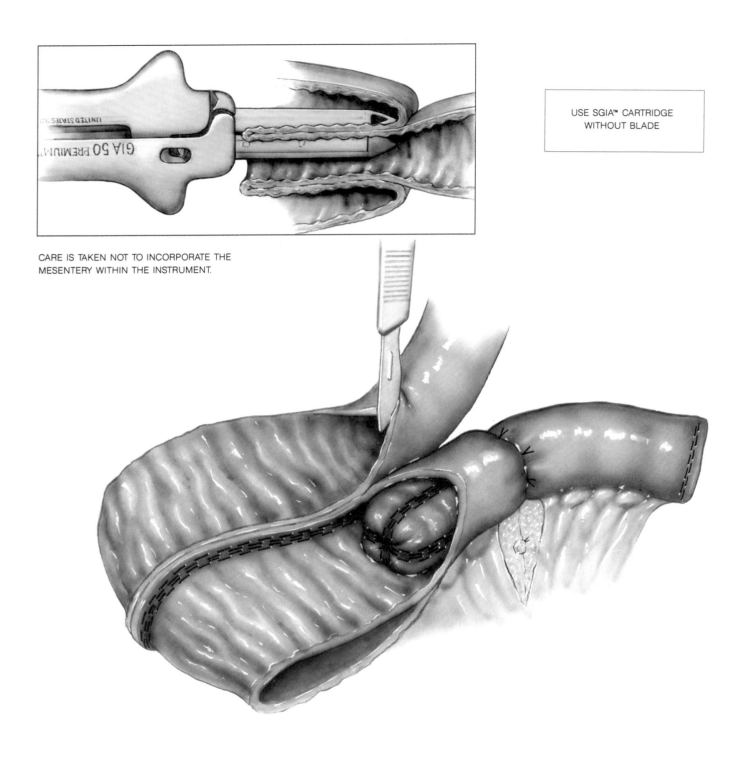

USE SGIA™ CARTRIDGE
WITHOUT BLADE

CARE IS TAKEN NOT TO INCORPORATE THE
MESENTERY WITHIN THE INSTRUMENT.

The shape of the nipple is maintained with anchoring U-shaped sutures of silk and three or four applications of the GIA™ instrument utilizing the SGIA™ loading unit. Insert the cartridge fork into the lumen of the nipple, thereby insuring that placement of the staple cross-span is intraluminal and the staple leg is extraluminal. This avoids any possibility of distorting a staple leg by the continual insertion and removal of a catheter.

In order to separate the afferent loop from the nipple of the efferent loop, incise the anterior wall of the afferent loop for a distance of 5 cm. Fold the flat bowel segment upon itself along its transverse axis apposing the serosal surfaces of the future pouch.

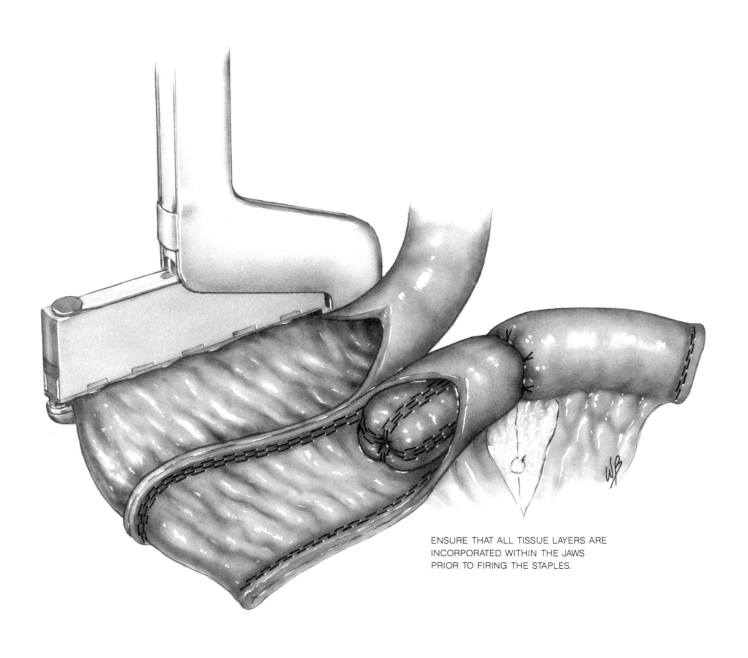

ENSURE THAT ALL TISSUE LAYERS ARE
INCORPORATED WITHIN THE JAWS
PRIOR TO FIRING THE STAPLES.

The lateral walls of the pouch are closed in an inverting fashion with the TA® 90 instrument. Approximate
the lateral pouch edges serosa to serosa with traction
sutures or Allis clamps. Slip the jaws of the instrument
around the tissue beneath the traction sutures or Allis
clamps. Close the instrument and fire the staples. Prior
to removing the instrument, use the instrument edge
as a cutting guide to excise the margin of tissue
protruding through the jaws. Repeat the procedure to
close the opposite lateral wall.

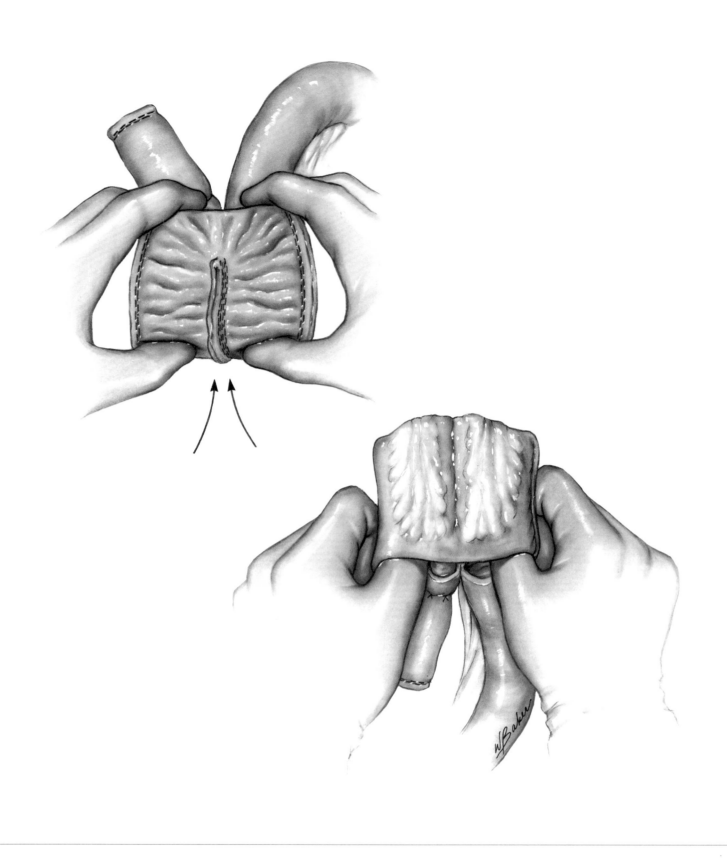

Following placement of the inverting staple lines, the pouch is turned right-side out to assume its final shape with the serosal surface as the outer aspect.

If desired, closure of the lateral walls can be performed in an everting manner.

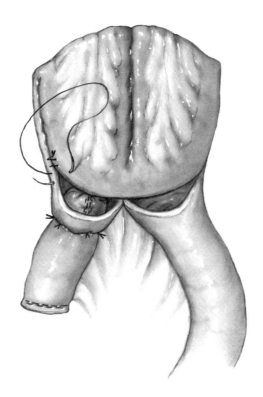

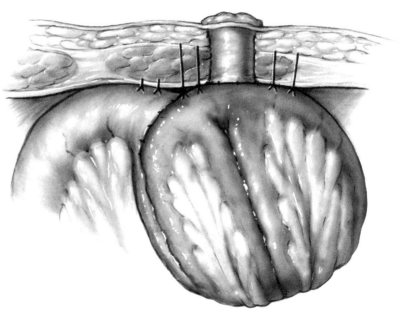

The anterior bowel edges extending between the nipple and afferent bowel are closed with a running suture of catgut and reinforced with interrupted sutures of silk. The nipple is also anchored externally with interrupted silk sutures. The pouch is positioned and secured, and the stoma is created.

Nipple competence is checked by injecting 100 ml. of saline into the pouch with a bowel clamp occluding the afferent limb. The pouch is emptied with a catheter introduced through the nipple.

The fascia and skin are closed in the usual manner with the DFS™ instrument and the PREMIUM® skin stapler.

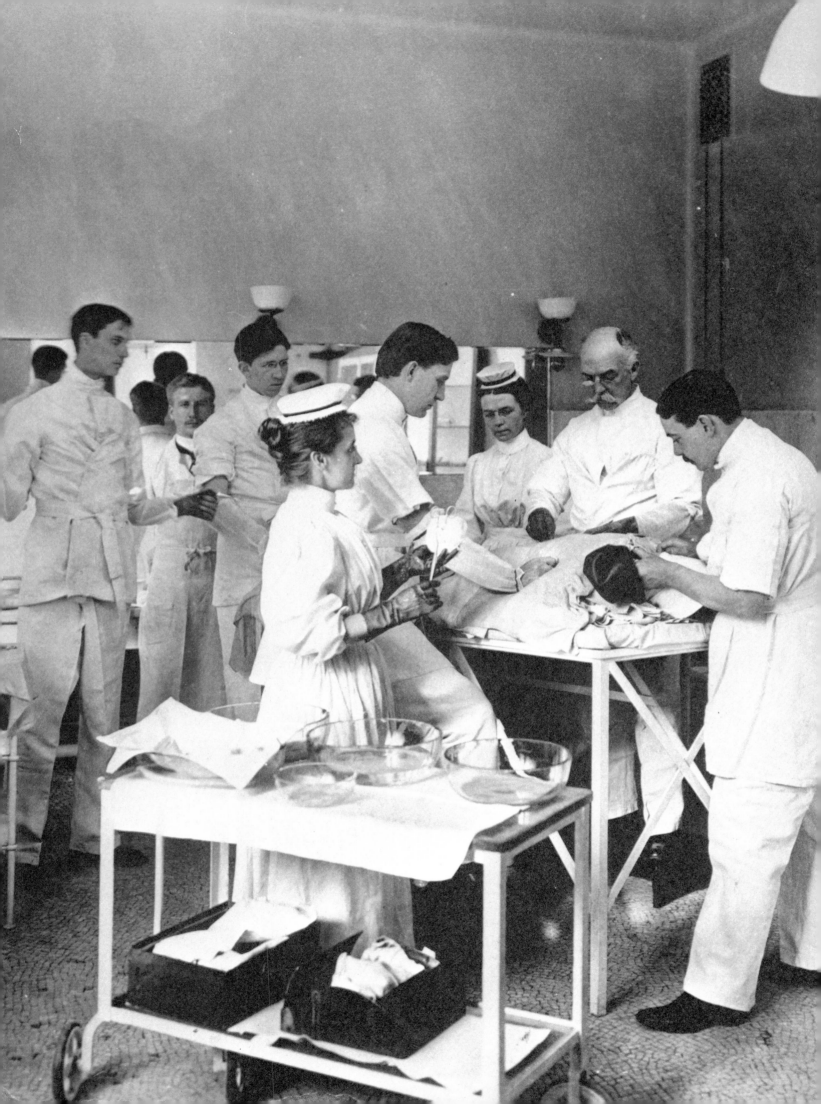

MISCELLANEOUS PROCEDURES

215

Cholecystectomy

Auto Suture® Instruments Used in a Cholecystectomy

See Cautions and Contraindications on page 236

INSTRUMENT	CLINICAL APPLICATION
PREMIUM SURGICLIP™ Clip Applier or SURGICLIP® Clip Applier	Ligation of the cystic artery and cystic duct. Ligation of accessory vessels.
DFS™ Instrument and PREMIUM® Skin Stapler	Closure of fascia and skin.

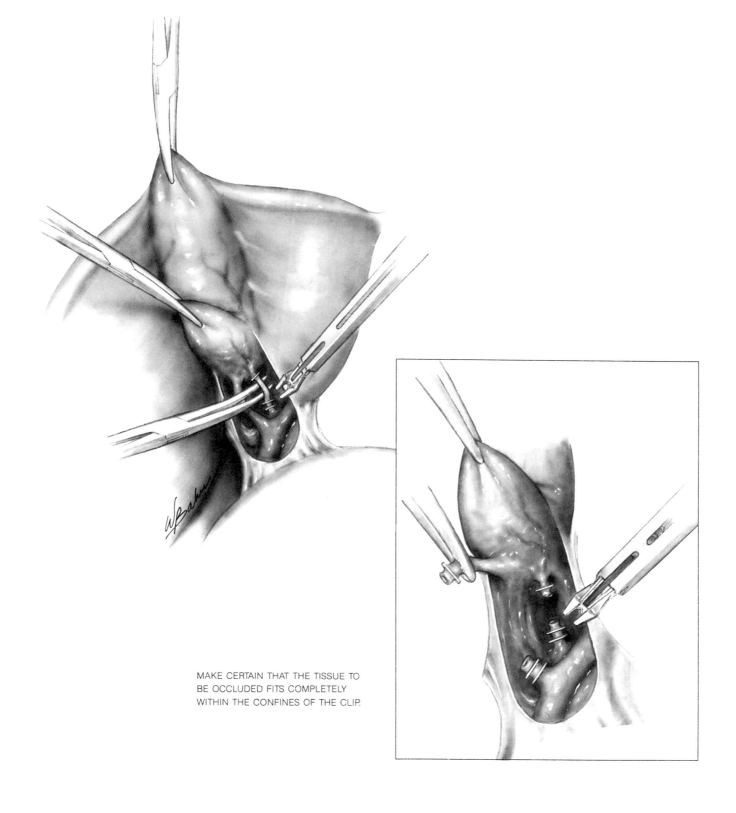

MAKE CERTAIN THAT THE TISSUE TO
BE OCCLUDED FITS COMPLETELY
WITHIN THE CONFINES OF THE CLIP.

The PREMIUM SURGICLIP™ clip applier is used to perform the cholecystectomy. The cystic artery is divided between two applications of the PREMIUM SURGICLIP™ clip applier leaving an adequate cuff on the proximal end. The cystic artery is doubly ligated on the patient side. The cystic duct is similarly ligated and divided at its junction with the common duct. Hemostasis of accessory vessels in the liver bed may be achieved using the PREMIUM SURGICLIP™ clip applier.

The fascia and skin are closed in the usual manner with the DFS™ instrument and the PREMIUM® skin stapler.

Choledochojejunostomy

Auto Suture® Instruments Used in a
Choledochojejunostomy with Gastrojejunostomy and Roux-en-Y

See Cautions and Contraindications on page 236

INSTRUMENT	CLINICAL APPLICATION
TA® 30 Instrument	Closure of the common bile duct.
GIA™ Instrument	Anastomosis of the cystic duct and hepatic duct. Anastomosis of the now common duct and the jejunum. Anastomosis of the jejunum to the stomach. Anastomosis of the proximal and distal jejunum for the Roux-en-Y.
TA® 90 Instrument	Closure of the common opening.
TA® 55 Instrument	Closure of the gastrojejunal stab wound. Closure of the jejunojejunal stab wound.
DFS™ Instrument and PREMIUM® Skin Stapler	Closure of fascia and skin.

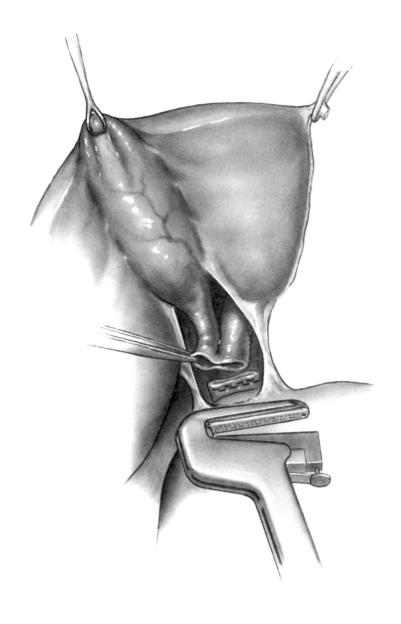

The TA® 30 instrument is used to close the common bile duct. Place the jaws of the instrument around the proximal common bile duct at the point of transection.

Close the instrument and fire the staples. Prior to removing the instrument, use the instrument edge as a cutting guide to transect the duct.

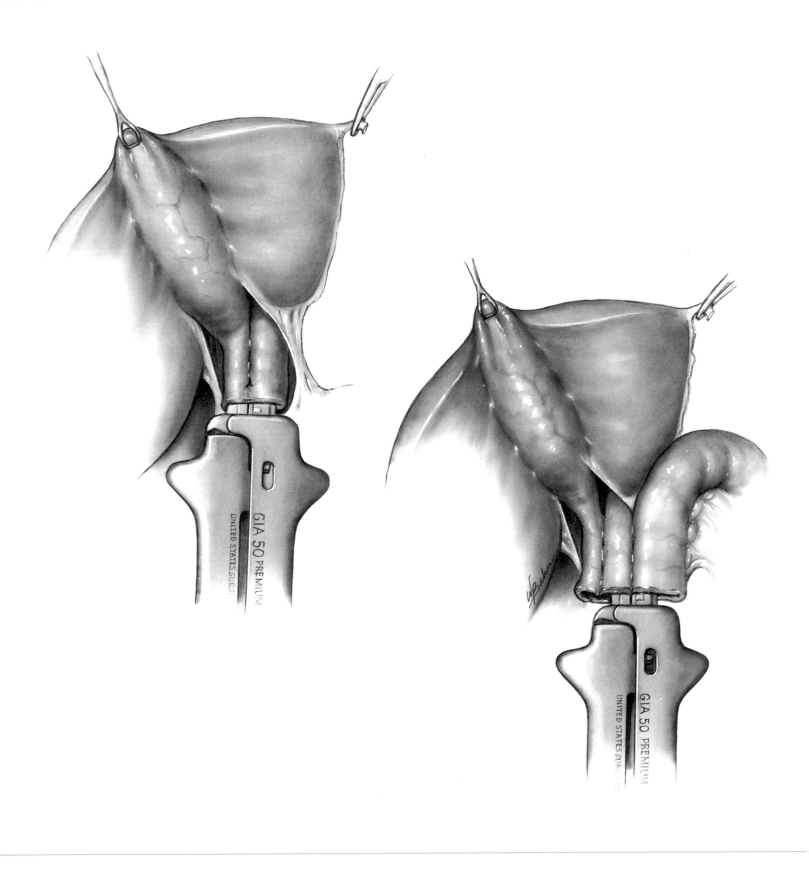

The GIA™ instrument is used to join the cystic and hepatic ducts, if both are of sufficient caliber to accommodate the instrument forks. Insert the anvil fork of the instrument into the lumen of the cystic duct and the cartridge fork into the lumen of the hepatic duct. Close the instrument and fire the staples.

A second application of the GIA™ instrument is used similarly to join the now common duct and the distal jejunum raised to the area through a rent in the mesocolon.

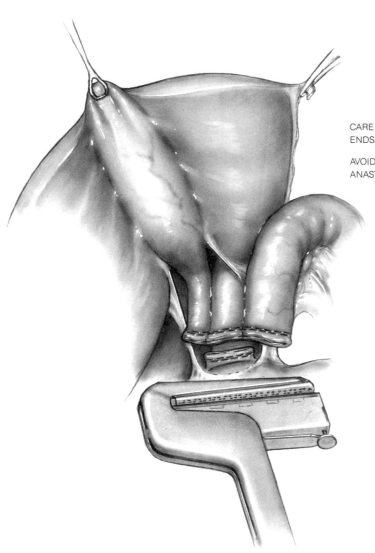

CARE MUST BE TAKEN TO OVERLAP THE
ENDS OF THE PREVIOUS STAPLE LINES.

AVOID DIRECT APPOSITION OF THE
ANASTOMOTIC STAPLE LINES.

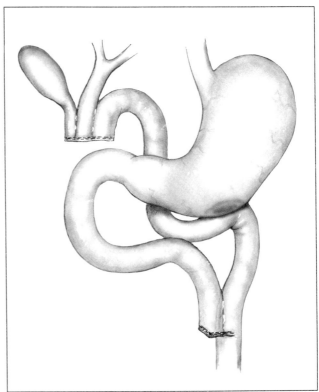

Inspect the anastomotic staple lines for hemostasis
prior to closure of the common opening with the
TA® 90 instrument.

The posterior retrocolic gastrojejunostomy and Roux-en-Y
jejunojejunostomy are performed as previously described.

The fascia and skin are closed in the usual manner
with the DFS™ instrument and the PREMIUM® skin
stapler.

Pancreaticocystogastrostomy

Auto Suture® Instruments Used in a Pancreaticocystogastrostomy

See Cautions and Contraindications on page 236

INSTRUMENT	CLINICAL APPLICATION
GIA™ Instrument	Creation of the gastrotomy. Anastomosis of the pancreatic cyst to the stomach.
TA® 90 Instrument	Closure of the gastrotomy.
DFS™ Instrument and PREMIUM® Skin Stapler	Closure of fascia and skin.

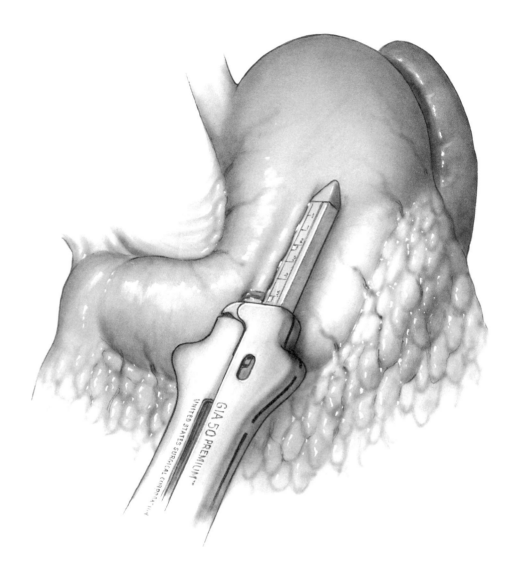

A gastrotomy is performed using the GIA™ instrument to incise the anterior wall of the stomach and secure hemostasis of the cut edges. Make a 1 cm. stab wound into the gastric wall at the level of the gastrotomy. Insert the anvil fork of the instrument into the lumen of the stomach and place the cartridge fork on the serosal surface. Close the instrument and fire the staples. Two double staggered staple lines are placed in the gastric wall and the knife blade in the instrument cuts an incision between them.

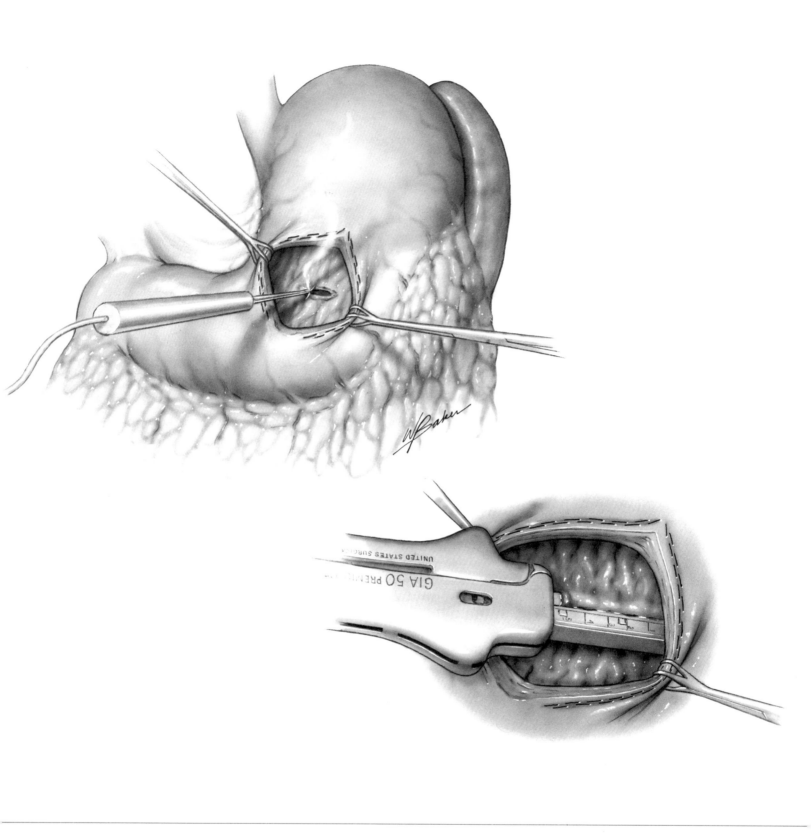

An opening is made into the cyst through the posterior gastric wall with electrocautery.

The GIA™ instrument is used to perform the pancreaticocystogastrostomy. Insert the anvil fork of the GIA™ instrument into the pancreatic cyst and the cartridge fork into the gastric lumen. Close the instrument and fire the staples. Two double staggered staple lines join the structures; simultaneously, the knife blade divides between the two double staple lines creating a stoma.

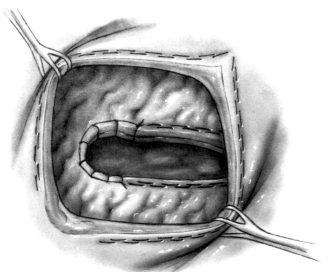

ALWAYS INSPECT THE ANASTOMOTIC STAPLE
LINES FOR HEMOSTASIS PRIOR TO
CLOSING THE GASTROTOMY.

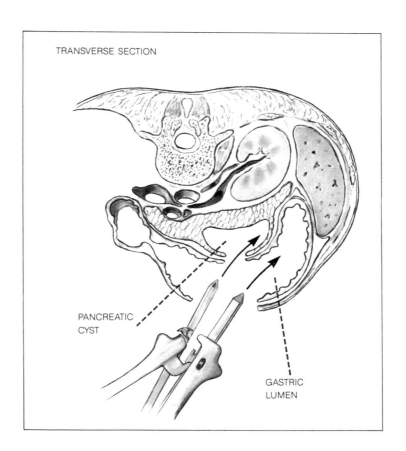

TRANSVERSE SECTION

PANCREATIC
CYST

GASTRIC
LUMEN

The stab wound edges are oversewn and the
anastomosis is inspected for hemostasis. The
gastrotomy is closed with the TA® 90 instrument.

The fascia and skin are closed in the usual manner
with the DFS™ instrument and the PREMIUM® skin
stapler.

Ileal Conduit

Auto Suture® Instruments Used in an Ileal Conduit Construction

See Cautions and Contraindications on page 236

INSTRUMENT	CLINICAL APPLICATION
LDS™ Instrument	Ligation and division of the mesenteric vessels.
GIA™ Instrument	Closure and transection of the proximal and distal ileum. Anastomosis of the proximal and distal ileum.
TA® 55 Instrument	Closure of the common opening. Closure of the proximal end of the ileal segment.
DFS™ Instrument and PREMIUM® Skin Stapler	Closure of fascia and skin.

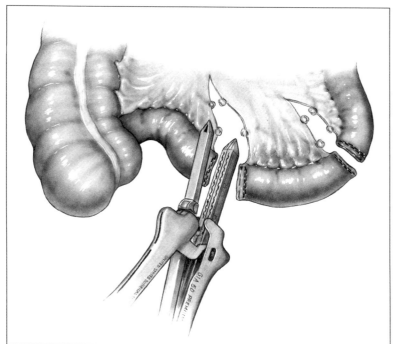

THE LDS™ INSTRUMENT MAY BE USED TO
LIGATE AND DIVIDE THE MESENTERIC VESSELS.

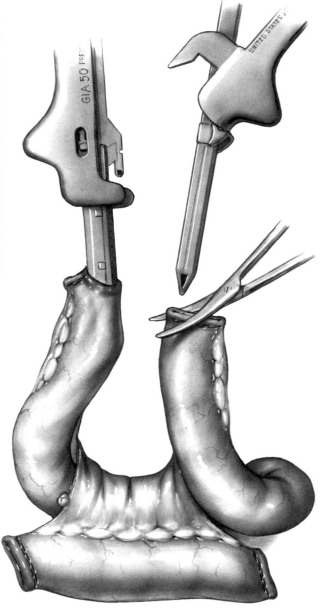

The ileal segment is identified beginning approximately
12-14 in. from the ileocecal valve and the incisions in
the mesentery are completed. The GIA™ instrument is
used to isolate the ileal segment. Place the instrument
around the ileum at the proximal point of transection.
Close the instrument and fire the staples. The instrument places two double staggered staple lines across
the ileum; simultaneously, a knife blade in the instru-

ment transects the ileum between the two double staple
lines. Reapply the GIA™ instrument to the distal end of the
ileal segment, 6-7 inches from the proximal staple line.

To re-establish bowel continuity, excise the
antimesenteric corner of both staple line closures.
Approximate the bowel and insert one fork of the
GIA™ instrument into each bowel lumen.

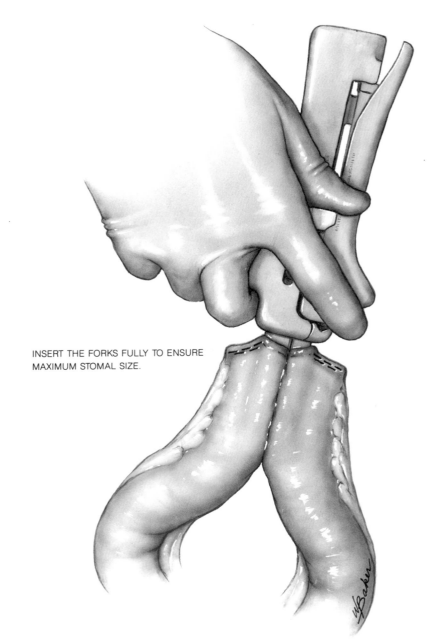

INSERT THE FORKS FULLY TO ENSURE MAXIMUM STOMAL SIZE.

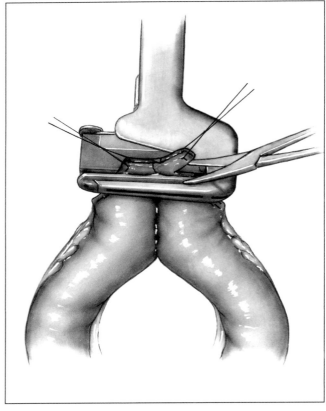

CARE MUST BE TAKEN TO OVERLAP THE ENDS OF THE PREVIOUS STAPLE LINES.

Align the bowel evenly on the GIA™ instrument forks. Close the instrument and fire the staples. Two double staggered staple lines join the bowel walls; simultaneously, the knife blade in the instrument divides between the two double staple lines creating a stoma.

Always inspect the anastomotic staple lines for hemostasis before closing the now common opening with the TA® 55 instrument.

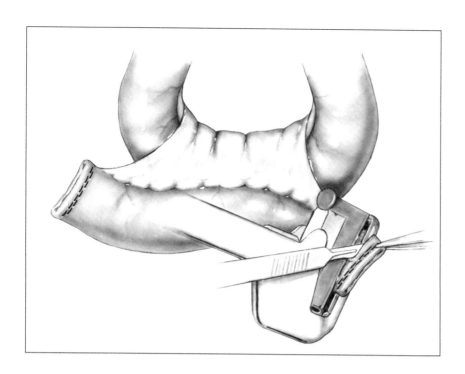

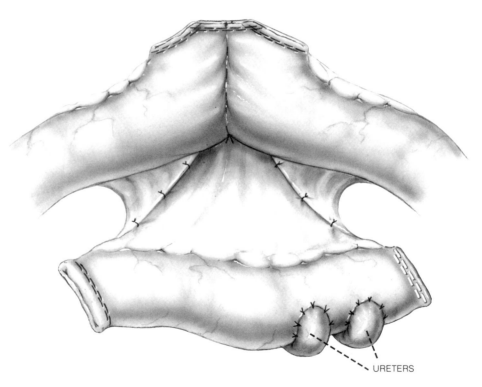

URETERS

The proximal end of the conduit is closed using the TA® 55 instrument with a POLYSORB™ 55 disposable loading unit. Place the instrument around the tissue just beneath the staple line closure. Close the instrument and fire the staples. Use the TA® 55 instrument edge as a cutting guide to excise the redundant tissue and staple line prior to removing the instrument.

The mesenteric hiatus between the ileoileostomy and the vascular pedicle of the ileal conduit is closed with interrupted sutures.

The uretero-ileal anastomosis is performed at the proximal end of the conduit.

The distal end of the ileal conduit is drawn through the external stoma created in the right abdominal wall. The staple line is excised and the edges of the ileal conduit are sutured to the skin with interrupted sutures.

The fascia and skin are closed in the usual manner with the DFS™ instrument and the PREMIUM® skin stapler.

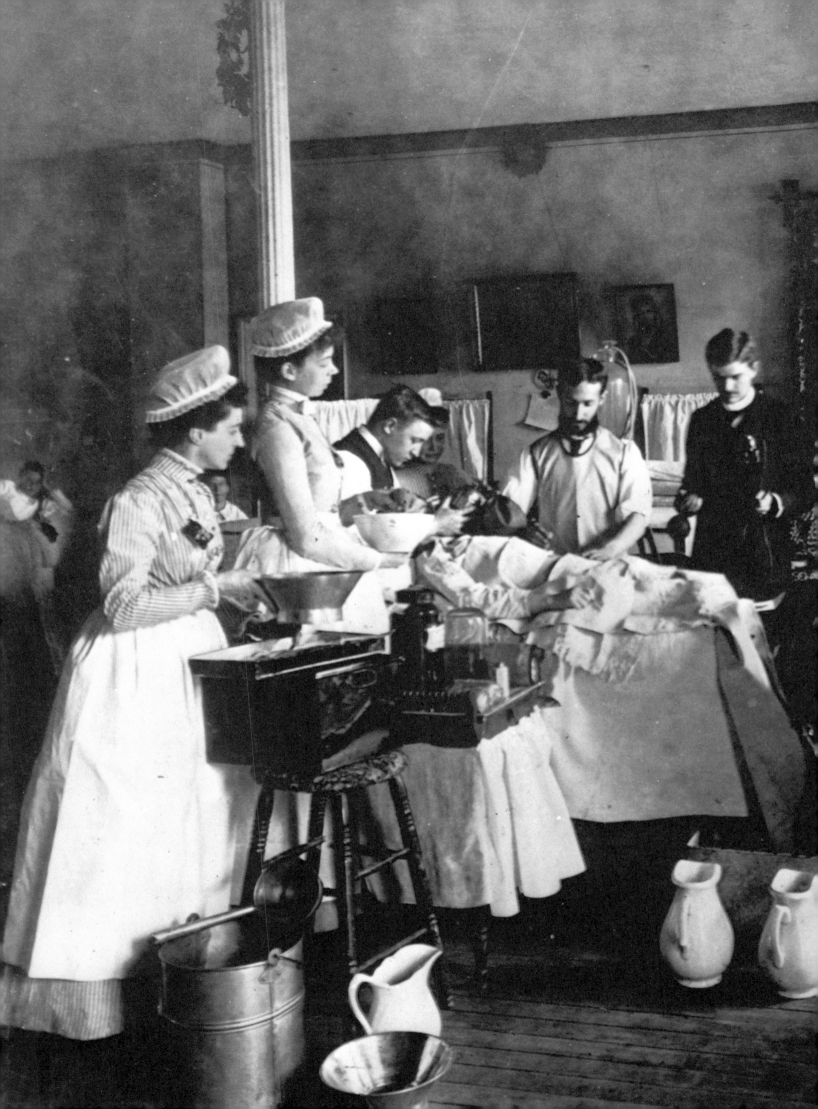

SKIN & FASCIA CLOSURE

Fascia Closure

Auto Suture® Instrument Used for
Fascia Closure

See Cautions and Contraindications on page 236

INSTRUMENT	CLINICAL APPLICATION
DFS™ Instrument	Fascia closure.

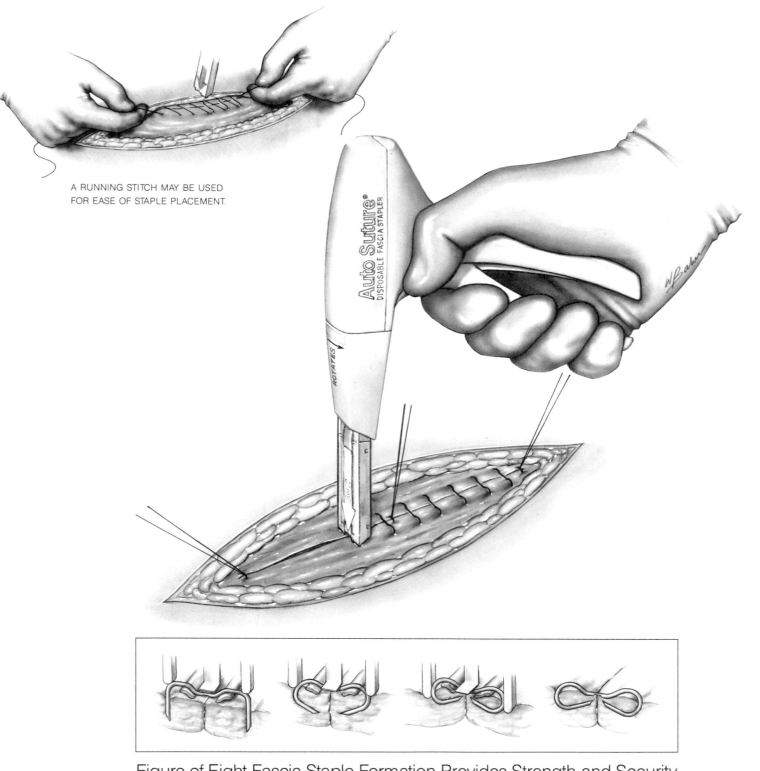

A RUNNING STITCH MAY BE USED
FOR EASE OF STAPLE PLACEMENT.

Figure-of-Eight Fascia Staple Formation Provides Strength and Security

The DFS™ instrument is used to close the fascia. Approximate the fascia with a running stitch or with traction sutures placed at 2-3 in. intervals. Place upward and outward traction on the sutures at the level of the tissue.

Press the cartridge firmly against the taut fascia with the cartridge held perpendicular and the locating arrow in the center of the incision. Squeeze the handle all the way until it stops and release. Move the cartridge forward and away.

Skin Closure

Auto Suture® Instrument Used for Skin Closure

See Cautions and Contraindications on page 236

INSTRUMENT	CLINICAL APPLICATION
PREMIUM® Skin Stapler	Skin closure.

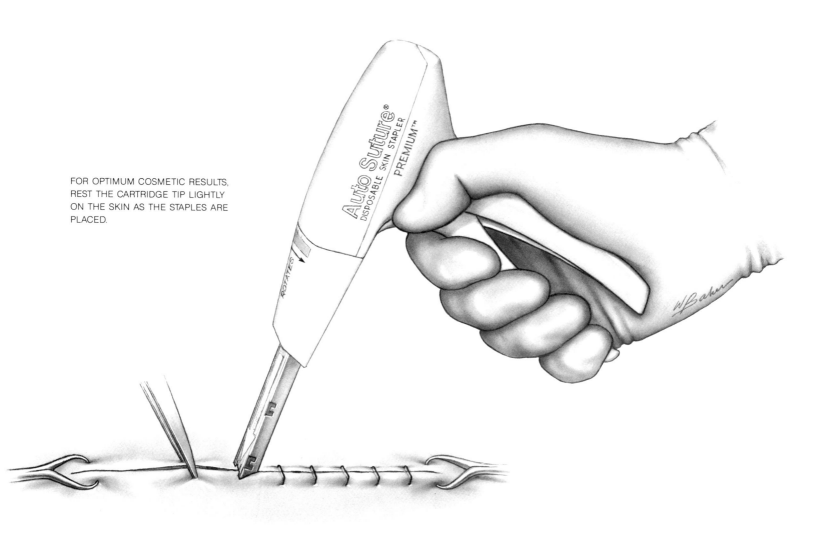

FOR OPTIMUM COSMETIC RESULTS,
REST THE CARTRIDGE TIP LIGHTLY
ON THE SKIN AS THE STAPLES ARE
PLACED.

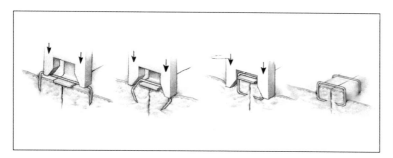

How Skin Staples Form and Hold Tissue

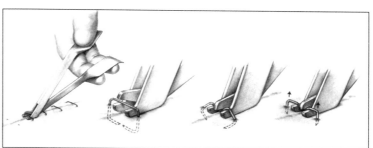

Simple Staple Removal From Skin

The PREMIUM® skin stapler provides excellent vision, positioning and control during staple placement.

Advance the staple into position at the tip of the cartridge by partially squeezing the handle. Place the cartridge lightly against the skin, at the angle of the bevel, with the locating arrow in the center of the incision. Complete the handle squeeze and release. This automatically disengages the staple.

The PREMIUM® skin stapler provides a rapid and precise skin closure with optimum cosmetic results.

CAUTIONS AND CONTRAINDICATIONS

The following cautions for the use of Auto Suture® surgical stapling instruments are recommended by surgeons experienced in the particular procedure discussed.

CAUTIONS IN PRIMARY TECHNIQUE

ESOPHAGOGASTRECTOMY

1. When the stomach is closed with two applications of the TA® 90 instrument, always leave the instrument in place after the second application and transect using the instrument edge as a cutting guide to obtain the proper distance between the staple line and the cut edge.
2. Allow a minimum of 10 cm. between the gastric staple line and the proximal end of the gastrotomy to ensure adequate blood supply to the tissue and anastomosis.
3. To ensure adequate blood supply to the tissue between the gastric edge and the anastomosis, allow a minimum of 2.5 cm. between the anastomotic and gastric staple lines.
4. Make sure that all gastric tissue layers are held firmly within the jaws of the purse string instrument and do not slip out as the purse string suture is placed. Use of an Allis clamp reduces this possibility.
5. Tie the purse string sutures securely, but not tightly, around the EEA™ instrument center rod. Ensure that the tissue is snug against the cartridge and anvil to reduce the possibility of bunching or overlapping of tissue as the instrument is closed.
6. As the instrument is closed, ensure that no extraneous tissue is incorporated between the cartridge and anvil.
7. Carefully check the circular specimen tissue remaining within the instrument cartridge for continuity of the purse string suture and all tissue layers.
8. Always inspect the anastomotic staple line for hemostasis prior to closure of the gastrotomy.
9. Make sure the stapled edges of the gastrotomy are held firmly within the TA® 55 instrument jaws and do not slip out as the instrument is closed. Use of traction sutures or Allis clamps reduces this possibility.

ESOPHAGECTOMY AND REVERSE GASTRIC TUBE

1. Oversew the gastric staple lines with inverting interrupted sutures or a continuous whip stitch.

ESOPHAGOGASTRECTOMY AND ISOPERISTALTIC GASTRIC TUBE

1. Oversew the gastric staple lines with inverting interrupted sutures or a continuous whip stitch.

ESOPHAGOGASTRECTOMY AND COLON REPLACEMENT

1. To ensure complete closure and transection of the segment of bowel to be isolated, make certain that the tissue does not extend past the zero calibration on the GIA™ instrument.
2. When the stomach is closed with two applications of the TA® 90 instrument, always leave the instrument in place after the second application and transect using the instrument edge as a cutting guide to obtain the proper distance between the staple line and the cut edge.
3. Perform anastomoses with the GIA™ instrument on the antimesenteric border of the bowel wall.
4. To ensure maximum stomal size, insert the forks fully into the lumina. Align the tissue edges evenly on the forks before closing the instrument.

5. Always inspect the anastomotic staple lines for hemostasis.
6. Closure of the esophagus and colonic stab wound is obtained with one application of the TA® 55 instrument applied obliquely. Take care to include the end staples of the anastomosis and all tissue layers within the instrument jaws.

PALLIATIVE SIDE-TO-SIDE ESOPHAGOGASTROSTOMY

1. To ensure maximum stomal size, insert the forks fully into the lumina. Align the tissue edges evenly on the forks before closing the instrument.
2. Always inspect the anastomotic staple lines for hemostasis prior to closure of the common stab wound.
3. When closing the common opening, take care to include the end staples of the anastomosis and all tissue layers within the TA® 55 instrument jaws.

COLLIS-NISSEN PROCEDURE

1. Oversew the gastric staple lines with inverting interrupted sutures or a continuous whip stitch.

ZENKER'S DIVERTICULECTOMY

1. Avoid strong traction on the diverticulum to prevent drawing normal esophagus into the instrument.

LIGATION OF ESOPHAGEAL VARICES

1. Tie the ligature snugly around the center rod of the EEA™ instrument.
2. Always inspect the anastomotic staple line for hemostasis prior to closing the gastrotomy.
3. Make sure the edges of the gastrotomy are held firmly within the TA® 55 instrument jaws and do not slip out as the instrument is closed. Use of traction sutures or Allis clamps reduces this possibility.

BILLROTH II

1. To ensure adequate blood supply to the tissue between the gastric edge and the anastomotic staple line, perform the gastrojejunostomy 2.5 cm. above the greater curvature and 2.5 cm. proximal to the gastric staple line.
2. Perform the anastomosis on the antimesenteric border of the jejunum.
3. To ensure maximum stomal size, insert the forks fully into the lumina. Align the tissue edges evenly on the forks before closing the instrument.
4. Always inspect the anastomotic staple lines for hemostasis following withdrawal of the forks.
5. When closing the common stab wound, take care to include the ends of the anastomotic staple lines, held in opposition, within the TA® 55 instrument jaws. Make sure that all tissue layers are held firmly within the instrument and do not slip out as the instrument is closed. The use of an Allis clamp at the midpoint reduces this possibility.

BILLROTH I

1. To prevent incorporation of LDS™ staples in the anastomosis, use the LDS™ instrument to within 2 cm. of the point of transection of the duodenum.
2. Allow a minimum of 3 cm. between the gastric staple line and the end of the gastrotomy to ensure adequate blood supply to the tissue.
3. To ensure adequate blood supply to the tissue between the gastric edge and the anastomosis, allow a minimum of 2.5 cm. between the anastomotic and gastric staple lines.
4. Make sure that all gastric tissue layers are held firmly within the jaws of the purse string instrument and do not slip out as the purse string suture is placed. Use of an Allis clamp reduces this possibility.
5. Tie the purse string sutures securely, but not tightly, around the EEA™ instrument center rod. Ensure that the tissue is snug against the cartridge and anvil to reduce the possibility of bunching or overlapping of tissue as the instrument is closed.
6. As the instrument is closed, ensure that no extraneous tissue is incorporated between the cartridge and anvil.
7. Carefully check the circular specimen tissue remaining within the instrument cartridge for continuity of the purse string suture and all tissue layers.
8. Always inspect the anastomotic staple line for hemostasis prior to closure of the gastrotomy.
9. Make sure the stapled edges of the gastrotomy are held firmly within the TA® 55 instrument jaws and do not slip out as the instrument is closed. Use of traction sutures or Allis clamps reduces this possibility.

TOTAL GASTRECTOMY AND ESOPHAGOJEJUNOSTOMY

1. To prevent incorporation of LDS™ staples in the anastomosis, use the LDS™ instrument to within 2 cm. of the points of transection.
2. Tie the purse string sutures securely, but not tightly, around the EEA™ instrument center rod. Ensure that the tissue is snug against the cartridge and anvil to reduce the possibility of bunching or overlapping of tissue as the instrument is closed.
3. As the instrument is closed, ensure that no extraneous tissue is incorporated between the cartridge and anvil.
4. Carefully check the circular specimen tissue remaining within the instrument cartridge for continuity of the purse string suture and all tissue layers.
5. Always inspect the anastomotic staple lines for hemostasis prior to transverse closure of the jejunotomy.
6. Make sure that all tissue layers of the jejunotomy are held firmly within the TA® 55 instrument jaws and do not slip out as the instrument is closed. Use of traction sutures or Allis clamps reduces this possibility.

TOTAL GASTRECTOMY AND JEJUNAL INTERPOSITION

1. To prevent incorporation of LDS™ staples in the anastomosis, use the LDS™ instrument to within 2 cm. of the points of transection.
2. Tie the purse string sutures securely, but not tightly, around the EEA™ instrument center rod. Ensure that the tissue is snug against the cartridge and anvil to reduce the possibility of bunching or overlapping of tissue as the instrument is closed.
3. As the instrument is closed, ensure that no extraneous tissue is incorporated between the cartridge and anvil.
4. Carefully check the circular specimen tissue remaining within the instrument cartridge for continuity of the purse string suture and all tissue layers.
5. Always inspect the anastomotic staple lines for hemostasis prior to transverse closure of the jejunotomy.
6. Make sure that all tissue layers of the jejunotomy are held firmly within the TA® 55 instrument jaws and do not slip out as the instrument is closed. Use of traction sutures or Allis clamps reduces this possibility.

PAULINO GASTRIC SUBSTITUTE

1. To ensure complete closure and transection of the bowel, make certain that the tissue does not extend past the zero calibration on the GIA™ instrument.
2. Perform the anastomoses on the antimesenteric border of the bowel wall.
3. Insert the forks fully into the lumina and align the tissue edges evenly on the forks before closing the instrument.
4. Care must be taken to incorporate the end staples of the previous application in subsequent applications to ensure continuity of the staple lines.
5. Always inspect the anastomotic staple lines for hemostasis following withdrawal of the forks.
6. When closing the common stab wound, take care to include the ends of the previous staple lines within the TA® 55 instrument jaws. Make sure that all tissue layers are held firmly within the instrument and do not slip out as the instrument is closed. The use of an Allis clamp at the midpoint reduces this possibility.
7. Tie the purse string sutures securely, but not tightly, around the EEA™ instrument center rod. Ensure that the tissue is snug against the cartridge and anvil to reduce the possibility of bunching or overlapping of tissue as the instrument is closed.
8. As the instrument is closed, ensure that no extraneous tissue is incorporated between the cartridge and anvil.
9. Always inspect the anastomotic staple line for hemostasis prior to closure of the jejunum.
10. Carefully check the circular specimen tissue remaining within the instrument cartridge for continuity of the purse string suture and all tissue layers.

HUNT LAWRENCE POUCH

1. To ensure complete closure and transection of the bowel, make certain that the tissue does not extend past the zero calibration on the GIA™ instrument.
2. Perform the anastomoses on the antimesenteric border of the bowel wall. Insert the forks fully into the lumina and align the tissue edges evenly on the forks before closing the instrument.
3. Care must be taken to incorporate the end staples of the previous application in subsequent applications to ensure continuity of the staple lines.
4. Always inspect the anastomotic staple lines for hemostasis following withdrawal of the forks.
5. Tie the purse string sutures securely, but not tightly, around the EEA™ instrument center rod. Ensure that the tissue is snug against the cartridge and anvil to reduce the possibility of bunching or overlapping of tissue as the instrument is closed.
6. As the instrument is closed, ensure that no extraneous tissue is incorporated between the cartridge and anvil.
7. Always inspect the anastomotic staple line for hemostasis prior to closure of the common stab wounds.
8. Carefully check the circular specimen tissue remaining within the instrument cartridge for continuity of the purse string suture and all tissue layers.
9. When closing the common stab wound, take care to include the ends of the previous staple lines within the TA® 55 instrument jaws. Make sure that all tissue layers are held firmly within the instrument and do not slip out as the instrument is closed. The use of an Allis clamp at the midpoint reduces this possibility.

GASTROSTOMY

1. The diameter of the tube must be wide enough to allow oversewing of the staple line.
2. Oversew the staple line with inverting interrupted sutures or a continuous whip stitch.

EXCISION OF GASTRIC WALL LESION

1. Make sure that all tissue layers are held firmly within the jaws of the instrument and do not slip out as the instrument is closed. Use of Babcock clamps reduces this possibility.

POSTERIOR RETROCOLIC GASTROENTEROSTOMY

1. Perform the anastomosis on the antimesenteric border of the jejunum.
2. To ensure maximum stomal size, insert the forks fully into the lumina. Align the tissue edges evenly on the forks before closing the instrument.
3. Always inspect the anastomotic staple lines for hemostasis following withdrawal of the forks.
4. When closing the common stab wound, take care to include the ends of the anastomotic staple lines, held in opposition, within the TA® 55 instrument jaws. Make sure that all tissue layers are held firmly within the instrument and do not slip out as the instrument is closed. The use of an Allis clamp at the midpoint reduces this possibility.

GASTRIC BYPASS

1. To ensure adequate blood supply to the tissue between the gastric staple line and the anastomotic staple line, perform the gastro-jejunostomy 2.5 cm. from the greater curvature and 2.5 cm. proximal to the gastric staple line.
2. Perform the anastomosis on the antimesenteric border of the jejunum.
3. When using the GIA™ instrument for the gastrojejunostomy, insert the forks 2-3 cm. into each lumen and align the tissue edges evenly on the forks.
4. Always inspect the anastomotic staple lines for hemostasis prior to closing the common stab wound.
5. When closing the common stab wound, take care to include the end staples of the anastomosis.

VERTICAL BANDED GASTROPLASTY

1. Ensure that the gastric tissue is evenly distributed between the EEA™ cartridge and anvil to avoid the possibility of tissue bunching as the instrument is closed.
2. The distance between the gastric window and the Angle of His should not exceed 9 cm.
3. Always inspect the staple line for hemostasis after creating the gastric window.
4. Carefully check the circular specimen tissue remaining in the instrument cartridge for continuity of all tissue layers.
5. When firing the TA 90 B™ instrument across the EEA™ instrument staple line, place the instrument so that the junction of these staple lines is as close to the lesser curvature as possible. This will avoid a large pouch segment at this staple line junction.

SILASTIC RING VERTICAL GASTROPLASTY

1. Apply the TA 90 BN™ instrument from the lesser curvature to the esophagogastric junction.
2. Be certain that the nasogastric tube is well within the confines of the instrument notch as the instrument is closed and fired.

HEINEKE-MIKULICZ PYLOROPLASTY

1. Make sure that all tissue layers are held firmly within the jaws of the instrument and do not slip out as the instrument is closed. Use of traction sutures reduces this possibility.

FINNEY PYLOROPLASTY

1. Before firing the instrument, make certain that the greater omentum is not incorporated between the GIA™ instrument forks.
2. Always inspect the anastomotic staple lines for hemostasis prior to closure of the stab wound.
3. When closing the stab wound, make sure that all tissue layers are held firmly within the jaws of the instrument and do not slip out as the instrument is closed. Use of traction sutures or Allis clamps reduces this possibility.
4. An anchor suture must be placed at the base of the anastomotic staple line to relieve tension on the anastomosis.

JABOULAY PYLOROPLASTY

1. Before firing the instrument, make certain that the greater omentum is not incorporated between the GIA™ instrument forks.
2. Always inspect the anastomotic staple lines for hemostasis prior to closure of the stab wound.

3. When closing the common stab wound, take care to include the ends of the anastomotic staple lines, held in opposition, within the TA® 55 instrument jaws. Make sure that all tissue layers are held firmly within the instrument and do not slip out as the instrument is closed. The use of an Allis clamp at the midpoint reduces this possibility.

END-TO-END ANASTOMOSIS

1. When creating an anastomosis using the principle of triangulation, care must be taken during the second and third application to include the ends of the previously placed staple lines within the instrument jaws.
2. Make sure that all tissue layers are held firmly within the jaws of the instrument and do not slip out as the instrument is closed. Use of traction sutures and an Allis clamp at the midpoint reduces this possibility.

FUNCTIONAL END-TO-END ANASTOMOSIS

1. To ensure complete closure and transection of the bowel, make certain that the tissue does not extend past the zero calibration on the GIA™ instrument.
2. Perform the enteroenterostomy on the antimesenteric borders of the apposed bowel. To ensure maximum stomal size, insert the forks fully into the lumina. Align the tissue edges evenly on the forks before closing the instrument.
3. Always inspect the anastomotic staple lines for hemostasis following withdrawal of the forks.
4. When closing the common opening, take care to include the ends of the previous staple lines within the TA® 55 instrument jaws. Make sure that all tissue layers are held firmly within the instrument and do not slip out as the instrument is closed. The use of an Allis clamp at the midpoint reduces this possibility.

BYPASS ENTEROENTEROSTOMY

1. Perform the anastomosis on the antimesenteric borders of the apposed bowel.
2. To ensure maximum stomal size, insert the forks fully into the lumina. Align the tissue edges evenly on the forks before closing the instrument.
3. Always inspect the anastomotic staple lines for hemostasis following withdrawal of the forks.
4. When closing the common stab wound, take care to include the ends of the anastomotic staple lines, held in opposition, within the TA® 55 instrument jaws. Make sure that all tissue layers are held firmly within the instrument and do not slip out as the instrument is closed. The use of an Allis clamp at the midpoint reduces this possibility.

DIVERTICULECTOMY

1. Avoid strong traction on the diverticulum to prevent drawing normal bowel into the instrument.

APPENDECTOMY

1. Do not attempt a primary appendectomy with the LDS™ instrument.

RESECTION OF TERMINAL ILEUM

1. To ensure complete closure and transection of the bowel, make certain that the tissue does not extend past the zero calibration on the GIA™ instrument.
2. Perform the enteroenterostomy on the antimesenteric borders of the apposed bowel. To ensure maximum stomal size, insert the forks fully into the lumina. Align the tissue edges evenly on the forks before closing the instrument.
3. Always inspect the anastomotic staple lines for hemostasis following withdrawal of the forks.
4. When closing the common opening and resecting the appendix, take care to include the ends of the previous staple lines within the TA® 55 instrument jaws. Make sure that all tissue layers are held firmly within the instrument and do not slip out as the instrument is closed. The use of an Allis clamp at the midpoint reduces this possibility.

BYPASS ILEOCOLOSTOMY

1. Perform the anastomosis on the antimesenteric borders of the apposed bowel.
2. To ensure maximum stomal size, insert the forks fully into the lumina. Align the tissue edges evenly on the forks before closing the instrument.
3. Always inspect the anastomotic staple lines for hemostasis following withdrawal of the forks.
4. When closing the common stab wound, take care to include the ends of the anastomotic staple lines, held in opposition, within the TA® 55 instrument jaws. Make sure that all tissue layers are held firmly within the instrument and do not slip out as the instrument is closed. The use of an Allis clamp at the midpoint reduces this possibility.

RIGHT HEMICOLECTOMY

1. To prevent incorporation of LDS™ staples in the anastomosis, use the LDS™ instrument to within 2 cm. of the point of transection of the ileum.
2. To ensure adequate blood supply to the tissue, perform the ileocolostomy 2.5 cm. from the proposed closure of the colon.
3. Tie the purse string sutures securely, but not tightly, around the EEA™ instrument center rod. Ensure that the tissue is snug against the cartridge and anvil to reduce the possibility of bunching or overlapping of tissue as the instrument is closed.
4. As the instrument is closed, ensure that no extraneous tissue is incorporated between the cartridge and anvil.
5. Carefully check the circular specimen tissue remaining within the instrument cartridge for continuity of the purse string suture and all tissue layers.
6. Always inspect the anastomotic staple line for hemostasis prior to closure of the transverse colon.
7. When closing the colon, make sure that all tissue layers are held firmly within the instrument and do not slip out as the instrument is closed. The use of traction sutures or Allis clamps reduces this possibility.

COLOCOLOSTOMY

1. To prevent incorporation of LDS™ staples in the anastomosis, use the LDS™ instrument to within 2 cm. of the proximal and distal points of transection.
2. To ensure adequate blood supply to the tissue, allow a minimum of 2.5 cm. between the end of the colotomy and the anastomotic site.
3. Tie the purse string sutures securely, but not tightly, around the EEA™ instrument center rod. Ensure that the tissue is snug against the cartridge and anvil to reduce the possibility of bunching or overlapping of tissue as the instrument is closed.
4. As the instrument is closed, ensure that no extraneous tissue is incorporated between the cartridge and anvil.
5. Always inspect the anastomotic staple line for hemostasis prior to transverse closure of the colotomy.
6. Carefully check the circular specimen tissue remaining within the instrument cartridge for continuity of the purse string suture and all tissue layers.
7. When closing the colotomy, make sure that all tissue layers are held firmly within the instrument and do not slip out as the instrument is closed. The use of traction sutures or Allis clamps reduces this possibility.

COLOSTOMY

1. To prevent incorporation of LDS™ staples in the anastomosis, use the LDS™ instrument to within 2 cm. of the point of transection of the proximal colon.
2. Tie the purse string suture snugly into the purse string notch on the anvil shaft. Ensure that the tissue is snug against the anvil to reduce the possibility of bunching or overlapping of tissue as the instrument is closed.
3. As the instrument is closed, ensure that no extraneous tissue is incorporated between the cartridge and anvil.
4. Always inspect the stoma for hemostasis.
5. Carefully check the circular specimen tissue remaining within the instrument for continuity of the purse string suture and all tissue layers.

LOW ANTERIOR RESECTION—END-TO-END ANASTOMOSIS

1. To prevent incorporation of LDS™ staples in the anastomosis, use the LDS™ instrument to within 2 cm. of the point of transection of the proximal colon and rectum.
2. Tie the purse string sutures securely, but not tightly. Ensure that the tissue is snug against the cartridge and anvil to reduce the possibility of bunching or overlapping of tissue as the instrument is closed.
3. As the instrument is closed, ensure that no extraneous tissue is incorporated between the cartridge and anvil.
4. Always inspect the anastomotic staple line for hemostasis.
5. Carefully check the circular specimen tissue remaining within the instrument cartridge for continuity of the purse string suture and all tissue layers.

LOW ANTERIOR RESECTION—SIDE-TO-SIDE ANASTOMOSIS

1. To ensure complete closure and transection of the colon, make certain that the tissue does not extend past the zero calibration on the GIA™ instrument.
2. Perform the anastomosis on the antimesenteric border of the colon. To ensure maximum stomal size, insert the forks fully into the lumina. Align the tissue edges evenly on the forks before closing the instrument.
3. Always inspect the anastomotic staple lines for hemostasis following withdrawal of the forks.
4. Closure of the rectum and stab wound is obtained with one application of the ROTICULATOR® 55 instrument. Take care to include the end staples of the anastomosis and all tissue layers within the instrument jaws.

DUHAMEL PROCEDURE

1. To prevent incorporation of LDS™ staples in the anastomosis, use the LDS™ instrument to within 2 cm. of the point of transection of the proximal colon and rectum.
2. To ensure complete closure and transection of the proximal colon, make certain that the tissue does not extend past the zero calibration on the GIA™ instrument.
3. Tie the purse string sutures securely, but not tightly. Ensure that the tissue is snug against the cartridge and anvil to reduce the possibility of bunching or overlapping of tissue as the instrument is closed.
4. As the instrument is closed, ensure that no extraneous tissue is incorporated between the cartridge and anvil.
5. Carefully check the circular specimen tissue remaining within the instrument cartridge for continuity of the purse string suture and all tissue layers.
6. To ensure complete colorectal anastomosis between the two circular openings, make certain the tissue does not extend past the zero calibration on the GIA™ instrument.
7. Always inspect all anastomotic staple lines for hemostasis prior to transverse closure of the colotomy.
8. When closing the colotomy, make sure that all tissue layers are held firmly within the instrument and do not slip out as the instrument is closed. The use of traction sutures or Allis clamps reduces this possibility.

ILEAL "J" POUCH

1. To ensure complete closure and transection of the ileum, make certain that the tissue does not extend past the zero calibration on the GIA™ instrument.
2. Perform the anastomoses on the antimesenteric border of the bowel wall.
3. Care must be taken to incorporate the end staples of the previous application in subsequent applications to ensure continuity of the staple lines.
4. Always inspect the anastomotic staple lines for hemostasis following withdrawal of the forks.
5. Tie the purse string sutures securely, but not tightly, around the EEA™ instrument center rod. Ensure that the tissue is snug against the cartridge and anvil to reduce the possibility of bunching or overlapping of tissue as the instrument is closed.
6. As the instrument is closed, ensure that no extraneous tissue is incorporated between the cartridge and anvil.
7. Always inspect the anastomotic staple line for hemostasis.
8. Carefully check the circular specimen tissue remaining within the instrument cartridge for continuity of the purse string suture and all tissue layers.

KOCK ILEAL RESERVOIR

1. Join the antimesenteric borders of the bowel to create the posterior wall of the pouch. With the last GIA™ instrument application, care must be taken to place the instrument forks well beyond the septum to ensure complete tissue closure.
2. Insert the cartridge fork into the lumen of the nipple to ensure that placement of the staple cross-span is intraluminal and the staple leg is extraluminal.
3. Make sure that all tissue layers are held firmly within the TA® 90 instrument jaws and do not slip out as the instrument is closed. The use of traction sutures or Allis clamps reduces this possibility.

CHOLECYSTECTOMY

1. Doubly ligate the cystic artery and cystic duct for added security.

CHOLEDOCHOJEJUNOSTOMY

1. Perform the anastomosis on the antimesenteric border of the jejunum.
2. Align the tissue edges evenly on the forks before closing the GIA™ instrument.
3. Always inspect the anastomotic staple lines for hemostasis following withdrawal of the forks.
4. When closing the common opening, take care to include the ends of the previous staple lines within the TA® 90 instrument jaws. Make sure that all tissue layers are held firmly within the instrument and do not slip out as the instrument is closed. The use of traction sutures or Allis clamps reduces this possibility.

PANCREATICOCYSTOGASTROSTOMY

1. Always inspect the anastomosis for hemostasis prior to closure of the gastrotomy.

ILEAL CONDUIT

1. To ensure complete closure and transection of the bowel, make certain that the tissue does not extend past the zero calibration on the GIA™ instrument.
2. Perform the enteroenterostomy on the antimesenteric borders of the apposed bowel. To ensure maximum stomal size, insert the forks fully into the lumina. Align the tissue edges evenly on the forks before closing the instrument.
3. Always inspect the anastomotic staple lines for hemostasis following withdrawal of the forks.
4. When closing the common opening, take care to include the ends of the previous staple lines within the TA® 55 instrument jaws. Make sure that all tissue layers are held firmly within the instrument and do not slip out as the instrument is closed. The use of an Allis clamp at the midpoint reduces this possibility.

IMPORTANT: Before using any Auto Suture® surgical stapling instrument, read carefully the current information booklet for that device. Cautions and contraindications for the use of some instruments may change periodically. The cautions and contraindications set forth in the current information booklet for a particular Auto Suture® surgical stapling instrument supercede the statements of cautions and contraindications appearing herein.

CAUTIONS AND CONTRAINDICATIONS FOR INSTRUMENT APPLICATION

AUTO SUTURE® POWERED DISPOSABLE LDS™ SURGICAL STAPLER

CAUTIONS:

1. Do not overload jaw. Incorporate only as much tissue as can be comfortably accommodated within the jaws of the powered disposable LDS™ instrument.
2. Be careful not to pull up on instrument when squeezing handle as this motion may tear tissue.
3. If instrument is ever fired without tissue in jaw, make certain closed staples are removed from metal portions of jaw (anvils) before instrument is fired again, or subsequent staples cannot form.
4. Inspect the ligation site to ensure proper application and that hemostasis has been achieved. If minor bleeding is observed after application, electrocautery or manual suturing may be necessary to complete hemostasis.
5. Do not autoclave.

READ ALL INSTRUCTIONS CAREFULLY.

CONTRAINDICATIONS:

1. Do not use the powered disposable LDS™ instrument on vessels that cannot be compressed to .75mm in thickness and 7.0mm in width.

AUTO SUTURE® TA PREMIUM™ 90 SURGICAL STAPLING INSTRUMENT AND DISPOSABLE LOADING UNITS

CAUTIONS:

1. Make sure disposable loading unit is properly placed. The tip of the anvil side must hook over the top of the front jaw of instrument. When closing the instrument jaws, approximating lever should be depressed completely until flush with instrument body (listen for audible click).
2. Press the retaining pin firmly into place to ensure proper alignment of the cartridge and anvil.
3. Do not fire instrument unless the jaws are closed, the tissue is compressed and the retaining pin is pressed into place.
4. Do not release the safety catch until you are ready to fire.
5. When firing the staples, the instrument handle must be squeezed as far as it will go.
6. Prior to removing, use the instrument edge as a cutting guide to ensure cutting at a proper distance from the staple line. Do not attempt to open instrument unless safety is in locked position.
7. After removing the instrument, always inspect the staple line for hemostasis. Minor bleeding may be controlled by means of electrocautery or manual sutures.
8. Remove disposable loading unit and discard. Never reuse any disposable parts.
9. The instrument should be routinely examined for wear or misalignment caused by mishandling or dropping.
10. In maintaining Auto Suture® surgical stapling instruments, an approved surgical instrument lubricant should be used after each cleaning.

READ ALL INSTRUCTIONS CAREFULLY.

CONTRAINDICATIONS:

1. If approximating lever does not close comfortably tissue is too thick and use is contraindicated.
2. Do not allow tissue to become compressed between the tissue gap block and the anvil, as this feature is designed to maintain the correct gap between the anvil and cartridge.
3. Do not use the 4.8 staple size on any tissue that compresses to less than 2mm in thickness. In such cases, the staple will not be tight enough to ensure hemostasis. However, the 3.5 staple size may be used on thinner tissue.
4. Do not use the 3.5 staple size on any tissue that compresses to less than 1.5mm in thickness. In such cases, the staple will not be tight enough to ensure hemostasis.
5. Do not use the 4.8 staple size on any tissue which cannot comfortably compress to 2mm thickness. In such cases, the tissue is too thick for the staple size.
6. Do not use the 3.5 staple size on any tissue which cannot comfortably compress to 1.5mm thickness. In such cases, the tissue is too thick for the staple size. However, the 4.8 staple size may be used.
7. Do not use the TA PREMIUM™ 90 instrument unless the organ to be stapled can be sufficiently mobilized to allow the retaining pin to move into position and, thus avoid the possibility of penetrating tissue with the pin. In procedures such as wedge resection of the lung, this contraindication does not apply.
8. The TA PREMIUM™ 90 instrument should not be used on tissue such as liver or spleen whose compressibility is such that closure of the instrument would be destructive.

AUTO SUTURE®
DISPOSABLE TA® 90
SURGICAL STAPLER

CAUTIONS:

1. When closing the instrument jaws, approximating lever must be depressed completely (listen for audible click). When the instrument is fully closed, the black indicator on the lever will not be visible.
2. Press the retaining pin firmly into place to ensure proper alignment of the cartridge and anvil.
3. Do not fire instrument unless the jaws are closed, the black lines are no longer visible, and the retaining pin is pressed into place.
4. Do not release the safety catch until you are ready to fire.
5. When firing the staples, the instrument handle must be squeezed as far as it will go.
6. Prior to removing, use the instrument edge as a cutting guide to ensure cutting at a proper distance from the staple line.
7. After removing the instrument, always inspect the staple line for hemostasis. Minor bleeding may be controlled by means of electrocautery or manual sutures.
8. Do not autoclave.

READ ALL INSTRUCTIONS CAREFULLY.

CONTRAINDICATIONS:

1. Do not use the 4.8 staple size on any tissue that compresses to less than 2mm in thickness. In such cases, the staple will not be tight enough to ensure hemostasis. However, the 3.5 staple size may be used on thinner tissue.
2. Do not use the 3.5 staple size on any tissue that compresses to less than 1.5mm in thickness. In such cases, the staple will not be tight enough to ensure hemostasis.
3. Do not use the 4.8 staple size on any tissue which cannot comfortably compress to 2mm thickness. In such cases, the tissue is too thick for the staple size.
4. Do not use the 3.5mm staple size on any tissue which cannot comfortably compress to 1.5mm thickness. In such cases, the tissue is too thick for the staple size. However, the 4.8 staple size may be used.
5. Do not use the disposable TA® 90 stapler unless the organ to be stapled can be sufficiently mobilized to allow the retaining pin to move into position and, thus, avoid the possibility of penetrating tissue with the pin. In procedures such as a wedge resection of the lung, this contraindication does not apply.
6. The disposable TA® 90 stapler should not be used on tissue such as liver or spleen whose compressibility is such that closure of the instrument would be destructive.

7. Do not fire the disposable TA® 90 stapler if the black indicator on the approximating lever is visible. If the approximating lever is not closed fully, the staples may not form properly when the handle is squeezed. Improperly formed staples may compromise the integrity of the staple line which may result in leakage or disruption.

AUTO SUTURE®
TA 90 B™ AND TA 90 BN™
SURGICAL STAPLING INSTRUMENTS
AND DISPOSABLE LOADING UNIT

CAUTIONS:

1. The TA 90 B™ and TA 90 BN™ instruments are intended for bariatric procedures only. Users of these instruments should be thoroughly trained in bariatric surgery and trained for specific postoperative management. Use of the instrument should be restricted to hospitals appropriately staffed and equipped to manage postoperative complications arising out of bariatric surgery.
2. Only use the TA 90 BN™ surgical stapling instrument when a channel is desired as the instrument does not staple completely across tissue.
3. Make sure the disposable loading unit is properly placed. The alignment posts must be within the alignment post slot in the instrument.
4. To ensure proper alignment of the cartridge and anvil, the retaining pin must be screwed firmly into the front jaw of the instrument and tightened as far as it will go. The groove at the back of the pin must be in the vertical position.
5. Do not fire the instrument unless the jaws are closed, the tissue is compressed and the retaining pin is screwed into place. The instrument jaws must be closed until the release lever is flush with the instrument body. Otherwise, the automatic safety mechanism will prevent the instrument from being fired.
6. Do not release the safety catch until you are ready to fire.
7. When firing the staples, the instrument handle must be squeezed as far as it will go. Return the safety to the locked position.
8. After removing the instrument, always inspect the staple line for hemostasis. Minor bleeding may be controlled by means of electrocautery or manual sutures.
9. Remove and discard the disposable loading unit. Never reuse any disposable part.
10. Never use the retaining pin as a lever to remove the cartridge.

FAILURE TO OBSERVE THE FOLLOWING CAUTIONS MAY RESULT IN INSTRUMENT MISALIGNMENT OR STAPLE MALFORMATION OR BOTH, WHICH MAY WEAKEN THE STAPLE LINE AND RESULT IN LEAKAGE OR DISRUPTION.

11. The instrument should be routinely examined for wear and for misalignment caused by mishandling or dropping.
12. In maintaining Auto Suture® surgical stapling instruments, an approved surgical instrument lubricant should be used after each cleaning.
13. Never interchange parts between a TA 90 B™ surgical stapling instrument, TA 90 BN™ surgical stapling instrument, or any other surgical stapling instruments.
14. Use only the 4.8 disposable loading unit with 4 equidistant rows of staples with the TA 90 B™ and TA 90 BN™ surgical stapling instruments. It is the only disposable loading unit equipped to fit these instruments.

READ ALL INSTRUCTIONS CAREFULLY.

CONTRAINDICATIONS:

1. Do not use the 4.8 disposable loading unit on any tissue which cannot comfortably compress to 2mm thickness. In such cases, the tissue is too thick for the staple size. Conversely, do not use on any tissue which compresses to less than 2mm in thicknesses.
2. Do not use either the TA 90 B™ or TA 90 BN™ surgical stapling instrument unless the organ to be stapled, i.e., the stomach, can be sufficiently mobilized to allow the retaining pin to move into position without penetrating tissue with the pin.
3. The TA 90 B™ and TA 90 BN™ instruments are to be used only on the stomach for bariatric surgery.

AUTO SUTURE®
TA PREMIUM™ 55
SURGICAL STAPLING INSTRUMENT
AND DISPOSABLE LOADING UNIT

CAUTIONS:

1. Make sure disposable loading unit is properly placed. The tip of the anvil side must hook over the top of the front jaw of instrument. When closing the instrument jaws, approximating lever should be depressed completely until flush with instrument body (listen for audible click).
2. Press the retaining pin firmly into place to ensure proper alignment of the cartridge and anvil.
3. Do not fire instrument unless the jaws are closed, the tissue is compressed and the retaining pin is pressed into place.
4. Do not release the safety catch until you are ready to fire.
5. When firing the staples, the instrument handle must be squeezed as far as it will go and released. The safety must then be returned to the locked position.
6. Prior to removing, use the instrument edge as a cutting guide to ensure cutting at a proper distance from the staple line.
7. After removing the instrument, always inspect the staple line for hemostasis. Minor bleeding may be controlled by means of electrocautery or manual sutures.
8. Remove disposable loading unit and discard. Never reuse any disposable part.
9. The instrument should be routinely examined for wear or misalignment caused by mishandling or dropping.
10. In maintaining Auto Suture® surgical stapling instruments, an approved surgical instrument lubricant should be used after each cleaning.

READ ALL INSTRUCTIONS CAREFULLY.

CONTRAINDICATIONS:

1. If approximating lever does not close comfortably tissue is too thick and use is contraindicated.
2. Do not allow tissue to become compressed between the tissue gap block and the anvil. The tissue gap block is designed to maintain the correct gap between the anvil and cartridge. If tissue is included in the tissue gap block staples may not form properly.
3. Do not use in the 4.8 staple size on any tissue that compresses to less than 2mm in thickness. In such cases, the staple will not be tight enough to ensure hemostasis. However, the 3.5 staple size may be used on thinner tissue.
4. Do not use the 3.5 staple size on any tissue that compresses to less than 1.5mm thickness. In such cases, the staple will not be tight enough to ensure hemostasis.
5. Do not use the 4.8 staple size on any tissue which cannot comfortably compress to 2mm thickness. In such cases, the tissue is too thick for the staple size.
6. Do not use the 3.5 staple size on any tissue which cannot comfortably compress to 1.5mm thickness. In such cases, the tissue is too thick for the staple size. However, the 4.8 staple size may be used.
7. Do not use the TA PREMIUM™ 55 instrument unless the organ to be stapled can be sufficiently mobilized to allow the retaining pin to move into position and thus, avoid the possibility of penetrating tissue with the pin. In procedures such as a wedge resection of the lung, this contraindication does not apply.
8. The TA PREMIUM™ 55 instrument should not be used on tissue such as liver or spleen where compressibility is such that closure of the instrument would be destructive.

AUTO SUTURE®
POLYSORB™ 55
DISPOSABLE LOADING UNIT

CAUTIONS:

1. Make sure disposable loading unit is properly placed. The retainer side of the cartridge must hook over the top of the front jaw of the instrument. When closing the instrument jaws, the approximating lever should be depressed completely until flush with instrument body (listen for audible click).
2. Press the retaining pin firmly into place to ensure proper alignment of the cartridge and retainer jaws.
3. Do not fire instrument unless the jaws are closed, the tissue is compressed and the retaining pin is pressed into place.
4. When firing the staples, the instrument handle must be squeezed as far as it will go and released. The safety must then be returned to the locked position.
5. Prior to removing, use the instrument edge as a cutting guide to ensure cutting at a proper distance from the staple line.
6. After removing the instrument, always inspect the staple line for hemostasis. Minor bleeding may be controlled by means of electro-autery or manual sutures.
7. Remove disposable loading unit and discard. Never attempt to reuse any disposable parts.
8. The instrument should be routinely examined for wear or misalignment caused by mishandling or dropping.
9. POLYSORB™ 55 disposable loading units are supplied sterile and are intended for one time use.

READ ALL INSTRUCTIONS CAREFULLY.

CONTRAINDICATIONS:

1. Do not use POLYSORB™ 55 disposable loading units on tissue which is too thick or too thin for the staple size. If tissue is too thick, the staple will not lock and closure will not be secure. Always check to be sure that all staples are locked. If tissue is too thin there will not be adequate tissue compression for hemostasis. Use the appropriate staple size as outlined in the chart below.

Do not use on tissue that compresses to less than, or which cannot comfortably compress to:		
Staple Size	**Inch**	**mm**
.060	.060	1.5
.110	.110	2.8
.170	.170	4.3
.200	.200	5.0

2. Do not use POLYSORB™ 55- .060 and .110 disposable loading units on the vaginal cuff, since the tissue is too thick. The .170 or .200 size may be used, depending on tissue thickness.
3. If the approximating lever does not close comfortably, or if the tissue gap block does not touch the retainer jaw when the approximating lever is closed, tissue is too thick and use of the cartridge is contraindicated.
4. Do not allow tissue to become compressed between the tissue gap block and the retainer jaw of the cartridge. The tissue gap block is designed to maintain the correct gap between the fastener and retainer jaws of the cartridge. If tissue is included in the tissue gap block, staples may not close properly.
5. Do not use the TA PREMIUM™ 55 instrument unless the organ to be stapled can be sufficiently mobilized to allow the retaining pin to move into position and thus avoid the possibility of penetrating tissue with the pin.
6. Do not use for radiographic markings, or where radiopacity is otherwise necessary or desired as Auto Suture® POLYSORB™ staples are radiotransparent.
7. Do not use where prolonged or permanent existence of a staple is desired.
8. Do not apply staples over an existing line of stainless steel or POLYSORB™ staples. Also do not apply stainless steel staples over an existing line of POLYSORB™ staples. In either case, staples may not close or form properly.
9. Do not use on tissue such as liver or spleen where compressibility is such that closure of the instrument would be destructive.
10. Do not use on the main stem or lobar bronchus as the tissue is brittle, and may prevent staples from closing properly.

DO NOT RESTERILIZE.

AUTO SUTURE®
DISPOSABLE TA® 55
SURGICAL STAPLER

CAUTIONS:

1. When closing the instrument jaws, approximating lever must be depressed completely (listen for audible click). When the instrument is fully closed, the black indicator on the lever will not be visible.
2. Press the retaining pin firmly into place to ensure proper alignment of the cartridge and anvil.
3. Do not fire instrument unless the jaws are closed, the black lines are no longer visible, and the retaining pin is pressed into place.
4. Do not release the safety catch until you are ready to fire.
5. When firing the staples, the instrument handle must be squeezed as far as it will go.
6. Prior to removing, use the instrument edge as a cutting guide to ensure cutting at a proper distance from the staple line.
7. After removing the instrument, always inspect the staple line for hemostasis. Minor bleeding may be controlled by means of electro-cautery or manual sutures.
8. Do not autoclave.

READ ALL INSTRUCTIONS CAREFULLY.

CONTRAINDICATIONS:

1. Do not use the 4.8 staple size on any tissue that compresses to less than 2mm in thickness. In such cases, the staple will not be tight enough to ensure hemostasis. However, the 3.5 staple size may be used on thinner tissue.
2. Do not use the 3.5 staple size on any tissue that compresses to less than 1.5mm in thickness. In such cases, the staple will not be tight enough to ensure hemostasis.
3. Do not use the 4.8 staple size on any tissue which cannot comfortably compress to 2mm thickness. In such cases, the tissue is too thick for the staple size.
4. Do not use the 3.5mm staple size on any tissue which cannot comfortably compress to 1.5mm thickness. In such cases, the tissue is too thick for the staple size. However, the 4.8 staple size may be used.
5. Do not use the disposable TA® 55 stapler unless the organ to be stapled can be sufficiently mobilized to allow the retaining pin to move into position and, thus, avoid the possibility of penetrating tissue with the pin. In procedures such as a wedge resection of the lung, this contraindication does not apply.
6. The disposable TA® 55 stapler should not be used on tissue such as liver or spleen whose compressibility is such that closure of the instrument would be destructive.
7. Do not fire the disposable TA® 55 stapler if the black indicator on the approximating lever is visible. If the approximating lever is not closed fully, the staples may not form properly when the handle is squeezed. Improperly formed staples may compromise the integrity of the staple line which may result in leakage or disruption.

AUTO SUTURE®
MULTIFIRE TA™
DISPOSABLE SURGICAL STAPLER

CAUTIONS:

1. The MULTIFIRE TA™ disposable surgical stapler is for multiple use up to 4 times during a SINGLE surgical procedure only. Do not resterilize after use.
2. The MULTIFIRE TA™ disposable surgical stapler is designed to be fully disposable and should not be fired more than 4 times during a SINGLE procedure: otherwise, staples may not form correctly. Improperly formed staples could compromise the integrity of the staple line which may result in leakage or disruption.
3. When closing the instrument jaws, the approximating lever must be depressed completely: listen for audible click. When the instrument is closed fully, the black markings on the lever will not be visible. If the approximating lever is not closed fully, the staples may not form properly when the handle is squeezed. Improperly formed staples may compromise the integrity of the staple line which may result in leakage or disruption.
4. Press the retaining pin firmly into place to ensure proper alignment of the cartridge and anvil. Failure to properly align the cartridge and anvil may result in improperly formed staples. Improperly formed staples may compromise the integrity of the staple line which may result in leakage or disruption.
5. Do not release the safety catch until you are ready to fire.
6. When firing the staples, the instrument handle must be squeezed as far as it will go. Failure to squeeze the handle as far as it will go may result in underformed staples. Improperly formed staples may compromise the integrity of the staple line which may result in leakage or disruption.
7. Prior to removing, use the instrument edge as a cutting guide to ensure cutting at a proper distance from the staple line.
8. After removing the instrument, always inspect the staple line for hemostasis. Minor bleeding may be controlled by manual sutures or electrocautery.
9. The safety catch should be replaced immediately after firing, and must be in the locked position during all reloading stops.

READ ALL INSTRUCTIONS CAREFULLY.

CONTRAINDICATIONS:

1. The MULTIFIRE TA™ stapler must be used only in a SINGLE surgical procedure and must not be resterilized after use for application in a second procedure. Use of one instrument in two procedures may cause serious infection and other serious complications.
2. The MULTIFIRE TA™ stapler should not be fired more than 4 times; otherwise, staples may not form correctly. Improperly formed staples may compromise the integrity of the staple line which may result in leakage or disruption.
3. If the approximating lever does not close comfortably the tissue is too thick and use of the instrument is contraindicated.
4. Do not use 3.5mm staple size on any tissue that compresses to less than 1.5mm in thickness. In such cases, the staple will not be tight enough to ensure hemostasis.
5. Do not use 4.8mm staple size on any tissue that compresses to less than 2.0mm in thickness. In such cases, the staple will not be tight enough to ensure hemostasis; however, the 3.5mm staple size may be used provided that the position lever closes comfortably.
6. Do not use the MULTIFIRE TA™ stapler unless the organ to be stapled can be mobilized sufficiently to allow the retaining pin to move into position and, thus, avoid the possibility of penetrating tissue with the pin. In procedures such as a wedge resection of the lung, this contraindication does not apply.
7. The MULTIFIRE TA™ stapler should not be used on tissue such as liver or spleen whose compressibility is such that closure of the instrument would be destructive.
8. Do not fire the MULTIFIRE TA™ stapler if the black markings on the approximating lever are visible. In such cases, the jaws are not closed fully and staples may not form properly.

AUTO SUTURE®
ROTICULATOR® 55
DISPOSABLE SURGICAL STAPLER

CAUTIONS:

1. When closing the instrument jaws, the positioning lever must be depressed completely (listen for audible click). When the instrument is closed fully, the black markings on the lever will not be visible. If the positioning lever is not closed fully, the staples may not form properly when the handle is squeezed. This may compromise the integrity of the staple line which may result in leakage or disruption.

2. Press the retaining pin firmly into place to ensure proper alignment of the cartridge and anvil. Failure to properly align the cartridge and anvil may result in improperly formed staples. This may compromise the integrity of the staple line which may result in leakage or disruption.

3. When the instrument head is in the desired position, check to see that the locking mechanism has been rotated fully clockwise and the black markings are aligned, otherwise the angle of the instrument head may change.

4. Do not release the safety catch until you are ready to fire.

5. When firing the staples, the instrument handle must be squeezed until it locks onto the safety. Failure to squeeze the handle as far as it will go may result in underformed staples. This may compromise the integrity of the staple line which may result in leakage or disruption.

6. Prior to removing, use the instrument edge as a cutting guide to ensure cutting at a proper distance from the staple line.

7. After removing the instrument, always inspect the staple line for hemostasis. Minor bleeding may be controlled by manual sutures or electrocautery.

8. Do not autoclave.

READ ALL INSTRUCTIONS CAREFULLY.

CONTRAINDICATIONS

1. If the positioning lever does not close comfortably, tissue is too thick and use of the cartridge is contraindicated.

2. Do not use the 3.5 staple size on any tissue that compresses to less than 1.5mm in thickness. In such cases, the staple will not be tight enough to ensure hemostasis.

3. Do not use the 4.8 staple size on any tissue that compresses to less than 2.0mm in thickness. In such cases, the staple will not be tight enough to ensure hemostasis. However, the 3.5 staple size may be used provided that the positioning lever closes comfortably.

4. Do not use the ROTICULATOR® 55 stapler unless the organ to be stapled can be mobilized sufficiently to allow the retaining pin to move into position and, thus, avoid the possibility of penetrating tissue with the pin. In procedures such as a wedge resection of the lung, this contraindication does not apply.

5. The ROTICULATOR® 55 stapler should not be used on tissue such as liver or spleen whose compressibility is such that closure of the instrument would be destructive.

6. Do not fire the ROTICULATOR® 55 stapler if the black markings on the positioning lever are visible. In such cases, the jaws are not fully closed and staples may not form properly. Improperly formed staples may compromise the integrity of the staple line which may result in leakage or disruption.

AUTO SUTURE®
TA PREMIUM™ 30
SURGICAL STAPLING INSTRUMENT

CAUTIONS:

1. Make sure disposable loading unit is properly placed. The tip of the anvil side must hook over the top of the front jaw of instrument. When closing the instrument jaws, approximating lever should be depressed completely until flush with the instrument body (listen for audible click).

2. Press the retaining pin firmly into place to ensure proper alignment of the cartridge and anvil.

3. Do not fire instrument unless the jaws are closed, the tissue is compressed and the retaining pin is pressed into place.

4. Do not release the safety catch until you are ready to fire.

5. When firing the staples, the instrument handle must be squeezed as far as it will go and released. The safety must then be returned to the locked position. Failure to do so may result in jamming the instrument.

6. Prior to removing, use the instrument edge as a cutting guide to ensure cutting at a proper distance from the staple line.

7. After removing the instrument, always inspect the staple line for hemostasis. Minor bleeding may be corrected by means of electrocautery or manual sutures.

8. Remove disposable loading unit and discard. Never reuse any disposable part.

9. The instrument should be routinely examined for wear or misalignment caused by mishandling or dropping.

10. In maintaining Auto Suture® surgical stapling instruments, an approved surgical instrument lubricant should be used after each cleaning.

READ ALL INSTRUCTIONS CAREFULLY.

CONTRAINDICATIONS:

1. If approximating lever does not close comfortably tissue is too thick and use contraindicated.

2. Do not allow tissue to become compressed between the tissue-gap block and the anvil. The tissue-gap block is designed to maintain the correct gap between the anvil and cartridge. If tissue is included in the tissue-gap block staples may not form properly. This may compromise the integrity of the staple line which may result in leakage or disruption.

3. Do not use the 4.8 staple size on any tissue that compresses to less than 2mm in thickness. In such cases, the staple will not be tight enough to ensure hemostasis. However, the 3.5 or V staple size may be used on thinner tissue.

4. Do not use the 3.5 staple size on any tissue that compresses to less than 1.5mm in thickness. In such cases, the staple will not be tight enough to ensure hemostasis. However, the V staple size may be used on thinner tissue.

5. Do not use the 4.8 staple size on any tissue which cannot comfortably compress to 2mm thickness. In such cases, the tissue is too thick for the staple size.

6. Do not use the 3.5 staple size on any tissue which cannot comfortably compress to 1.5mm thickness. In such cases, the tissue is too thick for the staple size. However, the 4.8 staple size may be used.

7. Do not use the V and V 3 staple size on any tissue that compresses to less than 1.0mm in thickness. In such cases, the staple will not be tight enough to ensure hemostasis.

8. Do not use the V and V 3 staple size on any tissue which cannot comfortably compress to 1.0mm thickness. In such cases the tissue is too thick for the staple size. However, the 4.8 or the 3.5 staple size may be used.

9. Do not use the TA PREMIUM™ 30 instrument unless the organ to be stapled can be sufficiently mobilized to allow the retaining pin to move into position and, thus, avoid the possibility of penetrating tissue with the pin. In procedures such as wedge resection of the lung, this contraindication does not apply.

10. The TA PREMIUM™ 30 instrument should not be used on tissue such as liver or spleen where compressibility is such that closure of the instrument would be destructive.

AUTO SUTURE®
DISPOSABLE TA® 30
SURGICAL STAPLER

CAUTIONS:

1. When closing the instrument jaws, approximating lever must be depressed completely (listen for audible click). When the instrument is fully closed, the black indicator on the lever will not be visible.
2. Press the retaining pin firmly into place to ensure proper alignment of the cartridge and anvil.
3. Do not fire instrument unless the jaws are closed, the black lines are no longer visible, and the retaining pin is pressed into place.
4. Do not release the safety catch until you are ready to fire.
5. When firing the staples, the instrument handle must be squeezed as far as it will go.
6. Prior to removing, use the instrument edge as a cutting guide to ensure cutting at a proper distance from the staple line.
7. After removing the instrument, always inspect the staple line for hemostasis. Minor bleeding may be controlled by means of electrocautery or manual sutures.
8. Do not autoclave.

READ ALL INSTRUCTIONS CAREFULLY.

CONTRAINDICATIONS:

1. Do not use the 4.8 staple size on any tissue that compresses to less than 2mm in thickness. In such cases, the staple will not be tight enough to ensure hemostasis. However, the 3.5 or V staple size may be used on thinner tissue.
2. Do not use the 3.5 staple size on any tissue that compresses to less than 1.5mm in thickness. In such cases, the staple will not be tight enough to ensure hemostasis. However, the V staple size may be used on thinner tissue.
3. Do not use the V staple size on any tissue that compresses to less than 1.0mm in thickness. In such cases, the staple will not be tight enough to ensure hemostasis.
4. Do not use the 4.8 staple size on any tissue which cannot comfortably compress to 2mm thickness. In such cases, the tissue is too thick for the staple size.
5. Do not use the 3.5mm staple size on any tissue which cannot comfortably compress to 1.5mm thickness. In such cases, the tissue is too thick for the staple size. However, the 4.8 staple size may be used.
6. Do not use the V staple size on any tissue which cannot comfortably compress to 1.0mm thickness. In such cases, the tissue is too thick for the staple size. However, the 4.8 or the 3.5 staple size may be used.
7. Do not use the V staple size on the aorta because of vessel thickness.
8. Do not use the disposable TA® 30 stapler unless the organ to be stapled can be sufficiently mobilized to allow the retaining pin to move into position and, thus, avoid the possibility of penetrating tissue with the pin. In procedures such as a wedge resection of the lung, this contraindication does not apply.
9. The disposable TA® 30 stapler should not be used on tissue such as liver or spleen whose compressibility is such that closure of the instrument would be destructive.
10. Do not fire the disposable TA® 30 stapler if the black indicator on the approximating lever is visible. If the approximating lever is not closed fully, the staples may not form properly when the handle is squeezed. Improperly formed staples may compromise the integrity of the staple line which may result in leakage or disruption.

AUTO SUTURE®
GIA 90 PREMIUM™
SURGICAL STAPLER AND
DISPOSABLE LOADING UNIT

CAUTIONS:

1. Prior to firing, lock lever must be closed (listen for audible click).
2. When firing, push-bar mechanism handle must be pushed all the way forward until it stops and immediately pulled back all the way.
3. When using the GIA 90 PREMIUM™ stapler for anastomosis, insert the forks fully into each lumen, and align the tissue edges equally on the forks. After firing, always inspect the anastomotic staple line for hemostasis. Minor bleeding may be controlled by means of manual sutures or electrocautery.
4. When applying the instrument across the tissue or inserting forks into the lumina of the organ to be anastomosed, make certain tissue edges are properly aligned on the forks.
5. Dispose of cartridge/push-bar mechanism immediately after each use. Never reuse any disposable parts.
6. When using the instrument more than once during the same case, be sure that the anvil is clear of tissue, blood and staples following each application.
7. When using in the abdomen, make sure no omental or mesenteric vessels are caught between the forks prior to locking the instrument. In such cases, the staples may not be tight enough to ensure hemostasis.
8. In maintaining Auto Suture® surgical stapling instruments, an approved surgical instrument lubricant should be used after each cleaning.

READ ALL INSTRUCTIONS CAREFULLY.

CONTRAINDICATIONS:

1. Do not use the instrument on any tissue that compresses to less than 1.5mm in thickness. In such cases, the staple will not be tight enough to ensure hemostasis.
2. In gynecological surgery, the instrument should not be used on the infundibulopelvic ligament or across the uterine vessels. The staples may not be tight enough to ensure hemostasis.
3. Do not used the instrument on any tissue that cannot comfortably compress to 1.5mm in thickness. In such cases, the tissue is too thick for the staple size.
4. The instrument should not be used on tissue such as liver or spleen where compressibility is such that closure of the instrument would be destructive.
5. Tissue such as the duodenum or stomach may be too thick for application of the GIA 90 PREMIUM™ and SGIA 90 PREMIUM™ disposable loading units and, therefore, tissue thickness should be carefully evaluated before firing. However, the GIA 90 PREMIUM™ disposable loading unit can be used on the stomach for anastomosis.
6. The SGIA 90 PREMIUM™ disposable loading unit places four parallel rows of staples. Never manually divide between the rows of staples. If division is desired, the GIA 90 PREMIUM™ disposable loading unit is recommended.
7. Do not fire the instrument if serial numbers on instrument halves do not match.

AUTO SUTURE®
GIA 50 PREMIUM™
SURGICAL STAPLER AND
DISPOSABLE LOADING UNIT

CAUTIONS:

1. Prior to firing, lock lever must be closed (listen for audible click).
2. When firing, push-bar mechanism handle must be pushed all the way forward until it stops and immediately pulled back all the way.
3. When using the GIA 50 PREMIUM™ stapler for anastomosis, insert the forks fully into each lumen, and align the tissue edges equally on the forks. After firing, always inspect the anastomotic staple line for hemostasis. Minor bleeding may be controlled by means of electrocautery or manual sutures.
4. When applying the instrument across the tissue or inserting forks into the lumina of the organ to be anastomosed, make certain tissue edges are properly aligned on the forks and do not extend below the "5 mark" at the proximal end of the instrument.
5. Dispose of cartridge/push-bar mechanism immediately after each use. Never reuse any disposable parts.
6. When using the instrument more than once during the same case, be sure that the anvil is clear of tissue, blood and staples following each application.
7. When used in the abdomen, make sure no omental or mesenteric vessels are caught between the forks prior to locking the instrument. In such cases, the staples may not be tight enough to ensure hemostasis.
8. In maintaining Auto Suture® surgical stapling instruments, an approved surgical instrument lubricant should be used after each cleaning.

READ ALL INSTRUCTIONS CAREFULLY.

CONTRAINDICATIONS:

1. Do not use the instrument on any tissue that compresses to less than 1.5mm in thickness. In such cases, the staple will not be tight enough to ensure hemostasis.
2. In gynecological surgery, the instrument should not be used on the infundibulopelvic ligament or across the uterine vessels. The staples may not be tight enough to ensure hemostasis.
3. Do not use the instrument on any tissue that cannot comfortably compress to 1.5mm in thickness. In such cases, the tissue is too thick for the staple size.
4. The instrument should not be used on tissue such as liver or spleen where compressibility is such that closure of the instrument would be destructive.
5. Tissue such as the duodenum or stomach may be too thick for application of the GIA 50 PREMIUM™ and SGIA 50 PREMIUM™ disposable loading unit and therefore tissue thickness should be carefully evaluated before firing. However, the GIA 50 PREMIUM™ disposable loading unit can be used on the stomach for anastomosis.
6. The SGIA 50 PREMIUM™ disposable loading unit places four parallel rows of staples. Never manually divide between the rows of staples. If division is desired, the GIA 50 PREMIUM™ disposable loading unit is recommended.
7. Do not fire the instrument if serial numbers on instrument halves do not match.

AUTO SUTURE®
DISPOSABLE GIA™ 50
SURGICAL STAPLER

CAUTIONS:

1. Prior to firing, lock lever must be closed (listen for audible click).
2. When firing, push-bar/knife assembly handle must be pushed all the way forward until it stops and immediately pulled back all the way.
3. When using these instruments for anastomosis, insert the forks fully into each lumen, and align the tissue edges equally on the forks. After firing, always inspect the anastomotic staple line for hemostasis. Minor bleeding may be controlled by means of electrocautery or manual sutures.
4. The instrument should not be used on tissue such as liver or spleen where compressibility is such that closure of the instrument would be destructive.

5. When used in the abdomen, make sure no omental or mesenteric vessels are caught between the forks prior to locking the instrument. In such cases, the staples may not be tight enough to ensure hemostasis.
6. When applying the instrument across the tissue or inserting forks into the lumina of the organ to be anastomosed, make certain tissue edges are properly aligned on the forks and do not extend below the "5cm" mark at the proximal end of the instrument.
7. Do not autoclave.

READ ALL INSTRUCTIONS CAREFULLY.

CONTRAINDICATIONS:

1. Do not use the instrument on any tissue that compresses to less than 1.5mm in thickness. In such cases, the staple will not be tight enough to ensure hemostasis.
2. Do not use the instrument on any tissue that cannot comfortably compress to 1.5mm in thickness. In such cases, the tissue is too thick for the staple size.
3. Tissue such as the duodenum or stomach may be too thick for transection with the disposable GIA™ 50 stapler and, therefore, tissue thickness should be carefully evaluated before firing. However, the disposable GIA™ 50 stapler can be used on the stomach for anastomosis.

AUTO SUTURE®
DISPOSABLE SGIA™ 50
SURGICAL STAPLER

CAUTIONS:

1. Prior to firing, lock lever must be locked closed (listen for audible click).
2. When firing, push-bar handle must be pushed all the way forward until it stops and immediately pulled back all the way.
3. After firing, always inspect the staple line for hemostasis. Minor bleeding may be controlled by means of electrocautery or manual sutures.
4. The instrument should not be used on tissue such as liver or spleen whose compressibility is such that closure of the instrument would be destructive.
5. When used in the abdomen, make sure no omental or mesenteric vessels are caught between the forks prior to locking the instrument. In such cases, the staples may not be tight enough to ensure hemostasis.
6. Do not autoclave.

READ ALL INSTRUCTIONS CAREFULLY.

CONTRAINDICATIONS:

1. Do not use the instrument on any tissue that compresses to less than 1.5mm in thickness. In such cases, the staple will not be tight enough to ensure hemostasis.
2. Do not use the instrument on any tissue that cannot comfortably compress to 1.5mm in thickness. In such cases, the tissue is too thick for the staple size.
3. Tissue such as the duodenum or stomach may be too thick for application of the disposable SGIA™ 50 stapler and, therefore, tissue thickness should be carefully evaluated before firing.

AUTO SUTURE®
MULTIFIRE GIA™ 50
DISPOSABLE SURGICAL STAPLER
AND DISPOSABLE LOADING UNIT

CAUTIONS:

1. The MULTIFIRE GIA™ disposable surgical stapler is for multiple use during a SINGLE surgical procedure only. Do not resterilize after use.
2. The MULTIFIRE GIA™ 50 disposable surgical stapler is designed to be fully disposable and should not be fired more than 4 times during a SINGLE procedure; otherwise, staples may not form correctly. This could compromise the integrity of the staple line which may result in leakage or disruption.
3. Prior to firing, lock lever must be closed (listen for audible click).
4. When firing, plastic handle must be pushed all the way forward until it stops and then pulled back all the way to open the instrument.

5. When using the MULTIFIRE GIA™ 50 surgical stapler for anastomosis, insert the forks fully into each lumen and align the tissue edges equally on the forks. After firing, always inspect the anastomotic staple line for hemostasis. Minor bleeding may be controlled by electrocautery or manual sutures.

6. When applying the instrument across the tissue or inserting forks into the lumina of the organ to be anastomosed, make certain tissue edges are properly aligned on the forks and do not extend below the "5 mark" at the proximal end of the instrument.

7. Dispose of cartridge immediately after use. Never reuse any disposable loading unit.

8. When using the instrument more than once during the same procedure, be sure that the anvil is clean of tissue, blood and staples following each application. Obstructions on the anvil when instrument is fired may cause improperly formed staples. This may compromise the integrity of the staple line which may result in leakage or disruption.

9. When used in the abdomen, make sure no omental or mesenteric vessels are caught between the forks prior to locking the instrument. In such cases, the staples may not be tight enough to ensure hemostasis.

READ ALL INSTRUCTIONS CAREFULLY.

CONTRAINDICATIONS:

1. Do not use the instrument on any tissue that compresses to less than 1.5mm in thickness. In such cases, the staple will not be tight enough to ensure hemostasis.

2. In gynecological surgery, the instrument should not be used on the infundibulopelvic ligament or across the uterine vessels. The staples may not be tight enough to ensure hemostasis.

3. Do not use the instrument on any tissue that cannot comfortably compress to 1.5mm in thickness. In such cases, the tissue is too thick for the staple size.

4. The instrument should not be used on tissue such as liver or spleen where compressibility is such that closure of the instrument would be destructive.

5. Tissue such as the duodenum or stomach may be too thick for the disposable loading unit and therefore tissue thickness should be carefully evaluated before firing. However, the MULTIFIRE GIA™ 50 disposable loading unit can be used on the stomach for anastomosis.

AUTO SUTURE®
EEA™ SURGICAL STAPLING INSTRUMENT AND DISPOSABLE LOADING UNIT

CAUTIONS:

1. The anvil portion of the EEA™ disposable loading unit contains a white cutting ring. The cutting ring is normally found to be seated flush within the anvil. Absence or dislocation of this ring can result in failure of the instrument to cut properly, or in malformation of the staples. Malformed staples may compromise the integrity of the staple line resulting in leakage or disruption.

Check for proper position of cutting ring by using the following diagram as guides:

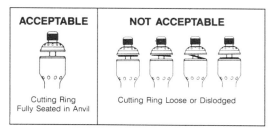

ACCEPTABLE	NOT ACCEPTABLE
Cutting Ring Fully Seated in Anvil	Cutting Ring Loose or Dislodged

If the ring is not properly seated, it can be returned to its proper position by pressing it into place, flush within the anvil.

2. To prevent premature discharge of staples, make certain safety is in locked position.

3. Make sure cartridge is properly seated and anvil is fully screwed down, otherwise staple malformation may result.

4. Purse string sutures must be placed no more than 2.5mm from the cut edges of the tissue to avoid excessive tissue within the closed anvil and cartridge which could cause staple malformation or leakage.

5. Cleaning the bowel too far from the cut edge could result in devascularizing the inverted tissue causing poor healing. The safety range for cleaning back is as follows: EEA™ 31 stapler-1.5cm, EEA™ 28 stapler-1.0cm, EEA™ 25 stapler-0.5cm.

6. Make certain that the section of tissue to be stapled is free from any metal clips, staples or sutures, otherwise the knife blade may not cut.

7. Make certain the space between cartridge and anvil is completely closed and the tissue compressed. The narrow black mark must be completely within the wider black marks prior to firing the staples. Failure to properly align the black marks may result in malformed staples.

8. Make certain firing stroke is completed as indicated by the markings on the rod, otherwise staples could malform.

9. After removing the instrument, always inspect the staple line for hemostasis. Minor bleeding may be controlled by means of electrocautery or manual sutures.

10. Dispose of anvil immediately after use. Dispose of cartridge following removal of the tissue specimens. To prevent injury, do not touch the circular knife covered by the white plastic ring. Never reuse any disposable parts.

11. The tissue specimens removed from the cartridge should be inspected to ensure that all tissue layers have been incorporated in the anastomosis. If the specimens are not complete, a small leak could result and cause narrowing.

12. In maintaining Auto Suture® surgical stapling instruments, an approved surgical instrument lubricant should be used after each cleaning.

13. Instruments should be routinely examined for wear or misalignment caused by mishandling or dropping.

14. Never interchange parts between EEA™ instruments. This could result in instrument malfunction.

15. Contact of the EEA™ disposable loading unit with mercuric chloride solutions may cause a chemical reaction and, therefore should be avoided.

READ ALL INSTRUCTIONS CAREFULLY.

CONTRAINDICATIONS:

1. Do not use the EEA™ 31, EEA™ 28 or EEA™ 25 disposable loading units on any tissue that compresses to less than 2.0mm in thickness in which case the staples will not be tight enough to ensure hemostasis.

2. Do not use the EEA™ 31, EEA™ 28 or EEA™ 25 disposable loading units on any tissue which cannot comfortably compress to 2.0mm in thickness. The instrument should not be used if unusual effort is required to turn the wing nut in order to align the black marks. The overly thick inverted tissue could be crushed when the cartridge and anvil are closed. Poor healing and narrowing of the anastomosis could result.

3. The EEA™ instrument should not be used if the tissue is stretched or thinned out by introducing a cartridge that is too large for the diameter of the structure. A leak may develop and lead to narrowing. Therefore, do not use the EEA™ 31 loading unit on any tubular tissue structure less than 31.6mm in diameter. Do not use the EEA™ 28 loading unit on any tubular structure less than 28.6mm in diameter. Do not use the EEA™ 25 loading unit on any tissue structure less than 25.0mm in diameter. A set of sizers is available to calibrate the size of the structures.

4. Do not use the EEA™ instrument unless there is sufficient tissue to allow proper inversion of tissue edges so staples can be placed securely. The purse string suture must be tied snugly around the center rod.

5. Never interchange disposable loading unit components. This may cause staple malformation.

AUTO SUTURE®
PREMIUM CEEA™
DISPOSABLE SURGICAL STAPLER

CAUTIONS:

1. The anvil portion of the PREMIUM CEEA™ disposable surgical stapler contains a white cutting ring. The cutting ring is normally found to be seated flush within the anvil. Absence or dislocation of the ring can result in failure of the instrument to cut properly, or in malformation of the staples. Malformed staples may compromise the integrity of the staple line resulting in leakage or disruption.

Check for proper position of cutting ring by using the following diagrams as guides:

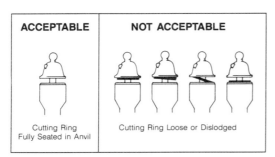

ACCEPTABLE	NOT ACCEPTABLE
Cutting Ring Fully Seated in Anvil	Cutting Ring Loose or Dislodged

If the ring is not properly seated, it can be returned to its proper position by pressing it into place, flush within the anvil.

2. Purse string sutures must be placed no more than 2.5mm from the cut edges of the tissue to avoid excessive tissue within the closed anvil and cartridge, which could cause staple malformation or leakage.

3. Cleaning the bowel too far from the cut edge could result in devascularizing the inverted tissue, causing poor healing. The safety range for cleaning back tissue is as follows:

PREMIUM CEEA™ 31 disposable surgical stapler - 1.5cm.

PREMIUM CEEA™ 28 disposable surgical stapler - 1.0cm.

PREMIUM CEEA™ 25 disposable surgical stapler - 0.5cm.

4. Make certain that the section of tissue to be stapled is free from any metal clips, staples or suture, otherwise the knife blade may not cut.

5. Make certain the space between cartridge and anvil is closed snugly and the tissue compressed. Inspect and assure that the green dot located in the tissue approximation indicator is partially visible within the black bars prior to firing the instrument. It is not necessary to have the entire green dot visible. If the green dot is not partially visible within the markings, staple malformation may occur which may compromise the integrity of the staple line resulting in leakage or disruption.

6. When opening the instrument prior to removal, do not turn wing nut more than three full turns, as this will cause the anvil shaft to rotate freely, thus hampering instrument removal.

7. After removing the instrument, always inspect the staple line for hemostasis. Minor bleeding can be controlled by means of electrocautery or manual sutures.

8. Dispose of anvils and trocars immediately after use. Following removal of tissue specimens from shaft, dispose of the instrument. To prevent injury, do not touch the circular knife.

9. The tissue specimens should be inspected to ensure that all tissue layers have been incorporated in the anastomosis. If the specimens are not complete, leakage and narrowing of the anastomosis could result.

10. Never reuse any components of disposable instruments.

11. Contact of the PREMIUM CEEA™ disposable surgical stapler with mercuric chloride solutions may cause a chemical reaction and, therefore, should be avoided.

12. Do not autoclave.

READ ALL INSTRUCTIONS CAREFULLY.

CONTRAINDICATIONS:

1. Do not use the PREMIUM CEEA™ disposable surgical stapler on any tissue that compresses to less than 2.0mm in thickness. In such cases, the staples will not be tight enough to ensure hemostasis.

2. Do not use the PREMIUM CEEA™ disposable surgical stapler on any tissue which cannot comfortably compress to 2.0mm in thickness. The instrument should not be used if unusual effort is required to turn the wing nut in order to visualize part of the green dot in the safety range area. Overly thick inverted tissue could be crushed when the cartridge and anvil are closed. Failure to create a stoma, poor healing, leakage, or narrowing of the anastomosis could result.

3. The PREMIUM CEEA™ disposable surgical stapler should not be used if the tissue is stretched or thinned out by introducing a cartridge that is too large for the diameter of the structure. Leakage and narrowing of the anastomosis could occur. Therefore, do not use the PREMIUM CEEA™ 31 disposable surgical stapler on any tubular tissue structure less than 31.6mm in diameter. Do not use the PREMIUM CEEA™ 28 disposable surgical stapler on any tubular tissue structure less than 28.6mm in diameter. Do not use the PREMIUM CEEA™ 25 disposable surgical stapler on any tubular tissue structure less than 25.0mm in diameter. A set of sizers is available to calibrate the size of the structures.

4. Do not use the PREMIUM CEEA™ disposable surgical stapler unless there is sufficient tissue to allow proper inversion of tissue edges so staples can be placed securely. The purse string suture must be tied snugly around the center rod.

AUTO SUTURE®
CURVED DISPOSABLE EEA™
SURGICAL STAPLER

CAUTIONS:

1. The anvil portion of the curved disposable EEA™ surgical stapler contains a white cutting ring. The cutting ring is normally found to be seated flush within the anvil. Absence or dislocation of this ring can result in failure of the instrument to cut properly, or in malformation of the staples. Malformed staples may compromise the integrity of the staple line resulting in leakage or disruption.

Check for proper position of cutting ring by using the following diagram as guides:

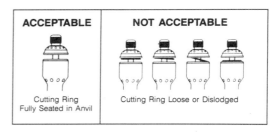

ACCEPTABLE	NOT ACCEPTABLE
Cutting Ring Fully Seated in Anvil	Cutting Ring Loose or Dislodged

If the ring is not properly seated, it can be returned to its proper position by pressing it into place, flush within the anvil.

2. Make sure anvil is fully screwed down, otherwise staple malformation may result.

3. Purse string sutures must be placed no more than 2.5mm from the cut edges of the tissue to avoid excessive tissue within the closed anvil and cartridge which could cause staple malformation or leakage.

4. Cleaning the bowel too far from the cut edge could result in devascularizing the inverted tissue causing poor healing. The safety range for cleaning back is as follows:

Curved disposable EEA™ 21 stapling instrument - 0.25cm.

5. Make certain that the section of tissue to be stapled is free from any metal clips, staples or sutures, otherwise the knife blade may not cut.

6. Make certain the space between cartridge and anvil is closed snugly and the tissue compressed. Assure that the green dot located in the tissue approximation indicator is partially visible within the black marks prior to firing the instrument. It is not necessary to have the entire green dot visible. If the green dot is not partially visible within the black marks, staple malformation may occur which may compromise the integrity of the staple line resulting in leakage or disruption.

7. After removing the instrument, always inspect the staple line for hemostasis. Minor bleeding may be controlled by means of electrocautery or manual sutures.
8. Dispose of anvil immediately after use. Following removal of the tissue specimens from cartridge, dispose of the instrument. To prevent injury, do not touch the circular knife covered by the white plastic ring.
9. The tissue specimens removed from the cartridge should be inspected to ensure that all tissue layers have been incorporated in the anastomosis. If the specimens are not complete, a small leak could result and cause narrowing.
10. Never reuse any components of disposable instruments.
11. Never interchange disposable anvils. This may cause staple malformation.
12. Contact of the curved disposable EEA™ stapler with mercuric chloride solutions may cause a chemical reaction and, therefore, should be avoided.
13. Do not attempt to turn wing nut if handles are squeezed as this may prevent reopening of the instrument.
14. Do not autoclave.

READ ALL INSTRUCTIONS CAREFULLY.

CONTRAINDICATIONS:

1. Do not use the curved disposable EEA™ stapler on any tissue that compresses to less than 2.0mm in thickness. In such cases, the staples will not be tight enough to ensure hemostasis.
2. Do not use the curved disposable EEA™ stapler on any tissue which cannot comfortably compress to 2.0mm in thickness. The instrument should not be used if unusual effort is required to turn the wing nut in order to visualize part of the green dot in the safety range area. Overly thick inverted tissue could be crushed when the cartridge and anvil are closed. Poor healing and narrowing of the anastomosis could result.
3. The curved disposable EEA™ stapler should not be used if the tissue is stretched or thinned out by introducing a cartridge that is too large for the diameter of the structure. A leak may develop and lead to narrowing. Therefore, do not use the curved disposable EEA™ 21 stapling instrument on any tubular tissue structure less than 20.9mm in diameter.
4. Do not use the curved disposable EEA™ stapling instrument unless there is sufficient tissue to allow proper inversion of tissue edges so staples can be placed securely. The purse string suture must be tied snugly around the center rod.

AUTO SUTURE® DISPOSABLE EEA™ SURGICAL STAPLER

CAUTIONS:

1. The anvil portion of the disposable EEA™ surgical stapler contains a white cutting ring. The cutting ring is normally found to be seated flush within the anvil. Absence or dislocation of this ring can result in failure of the instrument to cut properly, or in malformation of the staples. Malformed staples may compromise the integrity of the staple line resulting in leakage or disruption.

   Check for proper position of cutting ring by using the following diagram as guides:

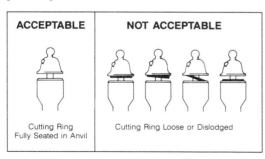

ACCEPTABLE	NOT ACCEPTABLE
Cutting Ring Fully Seated in Anvil	Cutting Ring Loose or Dislodged

   If the ring is not properly seated, it can be returned to its proper position by pressing it into place, flush within the anvil.
2. Purse string sutures must be placed no more than 2.5mm from the cut edges of the tissue to avoid excessive tissue within the closed anvil and cartridge which could cause staple malformation or leakage.

3. Cleaning the bowel too far from the cut edge could result in devascularizing the inverted tissue causing poor healing. The safety range for cleaning back is as follows.

   Disposable EEA™ 31 stapling instrument — 1.5cm.

   Disposable EEA™ 28 stapling instrument — 1.0cm.

   Disposable EEA™ 25 stapling instrument — .5cm.
4. Make certain that the section of tissue to be stapled is free from any metal clips, staples or sutures, otherwise the knife blade may not cut.
5. Make certain the space between cartridge and anvil is closed snugly and the tissue compressed. Assure that the green dot located in the tissue approximation indicator is partially visible within the black bars prior to firing the instrument. It is not necessary to have the entire green dot visible. If the green dot is not partially visible within the black bars, staple malformation may occur which may compromise the integrity of the staple line resulting in leakage or disruption.
6. After removing the instrument, always inspect the staple line for hemostasis.
7. Dispose of anvil immediately after use. Following removal of tissue specimens from cartridge, dispose of the instrument. To prevent injury, do not touch the circular knife covered by the white plastic ring.
8. The tissue specimens removed from the cartridge should be inspected to ensure that all tissue layers have been incorporated in the anastomosis. If the specimens are not complete, a small leak could result and cause narrowing.
9. Never reuse any components of disposable instruments.
10. Never interchange disposable anvils. This may cause staple malformation.
11. Contact of the disposable EEA™ stapler with mercuric chloride solutions may cause a chemical reaction and, therefore, should be avoided.

READ ALL INSTRUCTIONS CAREFULLY.

CONTRAINDICATIONS:

1. Do not use the disposable EEA™ stapler on any tissue that compresses to less than 2.0mm in thickness. In such cases, the staples will not be tight enough to ensure hemostasis.
2. Do not use the disposable EEA™ stapler on any tissue which cannot comfortably compress to 2.0mm in thickness. The instrument should not be used if unusual effort is required to turn the wing nut in order to visualize part of the green dot in the safety range area. Overly thick inverted tissue could be crushed when the cartridge and anvil are closed. Poor healing and narrowing of the anastomosis could result.
3. The disposable EEA™ stapler should not be used if the tissue is stretched or thinned out by introducing a cartridge that is too large for the diameter of the structure. A leak may develop and lead to narrowing. Therefore do not use the disposable EEA™ 31 stapling instrument on any tubular tissue structure less than 31.6mm in diameter. Do not use the disposable EEA™ 28 stapling instrument on any tubular tissue structure less than 28.6mm in diameter. Do not use the disposable EEA™ 25 stapling instrument on any tubular tissue structure less than 25.0mm in diameter. A set of sizers is available to calibrate the size of the structures.
4. Do not use the disposable EEA™ stapling instrument unless there is sufficient tissue to allow proper inversion of tissue edges so staples can be placed securely. The purse string suture must be tied snugly around the center rod.

AUTO SUTURE®
PURSE STRING INSTRUMENT

CAUTIONS:

1. Make certain the tissue structure is sufficiently mobilized to allow introduction of a straight needle in both directions.
2. Make certain the tissue structure is thick enough to fill the indentations in the jaws completely.
3. After removing instrument, inspect the lumen of the tissue structure for any possible cross stitching.
4. Instrument should be routinely examined for wear or misalignment.

CONTRAINDICATIONS:

1. Use of the AUTO SUTURE® Purse String instrument and placement of purse string sutures on friable tissue may be contraindicated.

AUTO SUTURE®
S-EEA™ SIZERS

CAUTIONS:

1. Lubricate sizer prior to introduction.
2. Make certain sizer head fits snugly without dilating the tissue.

AUTO SUTURE®
SURGICLIP® CLIP APPLIER

CAUTIONS:

1. Make certain a clip is positioned in the applying jaws before use.
2. Do not squeeze the handles before the jaws are placed around the tissue, as this will cause the clip to close and disengage prematurely.
3. Squeeze handles together firmly as far as they will go. Failure to squeeze the handles completely can result in clip malformation and possible bleeding.
4. Make certain that the tissue to be occluded fits completely within the confines of the clip or bleeding may result.
5. Some surgeons believe stainless steel or titanium should not be used in the brain.
6. Inspect the ligation site to ensure proper application and that hemostasis has been achieved. If minor bleeding is observed after application, electrocautery or placement of suture may be necessary to complete hemostasis.

READ ALL INSTRUCTIONS CAREFULLY.

CONTRAINDICATIONS:

1. Do not use these clips on the carotid artery, renal artery, iliac artery, and other vessels on which metal ligating clips would not normally be used.

AUTO SUTURE®
PREMIUM® AND DFS™
DISPOSABLE SKIN AND FASCIA STAPLERS

CAUTIONS:

1. PREMIUM® & DFS™ staplers are supplied sterile and are intended for one time use only. Do Not Autoclave.

READ ALL INSTRUCTIONS CAREFULLY.

CONTRAINDICATIONS:

1. Staples can be applied directly over bone or viscera; however, during application there must be a distance of not less than 6.5mm (slightly more than ¼") from the surface of the skin or fascia to the underlying bone, vessel, or viscera. When using the regular skin staple, the distance required can be slightly less, but at least 4.5mm. If these distances cannot be obtained by lifting the skin or fascia prior to application, use of skin or fascia staples is contraindicated.

AUTO SUTURE®
PREMIUM®
DISPOSABLE SKIN STAPLER REMOVER

CAUTION:

1. Slip lower jaws of PREMIUM® skin staple remover under staple. Make certain both tips are under the staple.

REFERENCES

Chassin J.L.: Operative Strategy in General Surgery—An Expositive Atlas. New York, Springer—Verlag, 1980.

Corman M.L.: Colon and Rectal Surgery, 2nd ed. Philadelphia, J.B. Lippincott Company, 1988.

Kremer K., Lierse W., Schreiber H.W.: Chirurgische Operationslehre— Ösophagus, Magen, Duodenum. Stuttgart, Georg Thieme Verlag, 1987.

Nelson R.L., Nyhus L.M.: Surgery of the Small Intestine. Norwalk, CT, Appleton-Century-Crofts, 1987.

Nyhus L.M., Baker R.J.: Mastery of Surgery. Boston, Little, Brown and Company, 1984.

Nyhus L.M., Wastell, C.: Surgery of the Stomach and Duodenum. Boston, Little, Brown and Company, 1986.

Ravitch M.M., Steichen F.M.: Atlas of General Thoracic Surgery. Philadelphia, W.B. Saunders Company, 1988.

Ravitch M.M., Steichen F.M.: Principles and Practice of Surgical Stapling. Chicago, Year Book Medical Publishers, 1987.

Ravitch M.M., Steichen F.M. (eds.): The Surgical Clinics of North America, Vol. 64, No. 3. Philadelphia, W.B. Saunders Company, June 1984.

Schwartz S.I., Ellis H.: Maingot's Abdominal Operations, 8th ed. Norwalk, CT, Appleton-Century-Crofts, 1985.

Shackelford R.T., Zuidema G.D. (eds.): Surgery of the Alimentary Tract, 2nd ed. Philadelphia, W.B. Saunders Company, 1981.

Shires G.T., et al (eds.): Advances in Surgery, Vol. 17. Chicago, Year Book Medical Publishers, 1984.

Steichen F.M., Ravitch M.M.: Stapling in Surgery. Chicago, Year Book Medical Publishers, 1984.

Ulrich B.: Chirurgische Gastroenterologie mit Interdisziplinären Gesprächen, Klammernaht—Technik. Hameln, TM-Verlag, October, 1986.

Ulrich B., Winter J.: Klammernahttechnik in Thorax und Abdomen. Stuttgart, Ferdinand Enke Verlag, 1986.

Welter R., Patel J.C.: Chirurgie Mécanique Digestive. Paris, Masson, 1985.

Wheeless C.R. Jr.: Atlas of Pelvic Surgery, 2nd ed. Philadelphia, Lea & Febiger, 1988.

Zollinger R.M. Jr., Zollinger R.M.: Atlas of Surgical Operations, 6th ed. New York, Macmillan Publishing Company, 1988.